Emergency Medical Responder

Your First Response in Emergency Care

Student Workbook

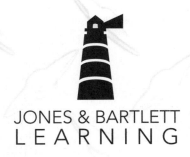

JONES & BARTLETT
LEARNING

World Headquarters
Jones & Bartlett Learning
5 Wall Street
Burlington, MA 01803
978-443-5000
info@jblearning.com
www.jblearning.com

Substantial discounts on bulk quantities of Jones & Bartlett Learning publications are available to corporations, professional associations, and other qualified organizations. For details and specific discount information, contact the special sales department at Jones & Bartlett Learning via the below contact information or send an email to specialsales@jblearning.com.

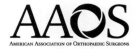

AMERICAN ASSOCIATION OF ORTHOPAEDIC SURGEONS

Jones & Bartlett Learning books and products are available through most bookstores and online booksellers. To contact Jones & Bartlett Learning directly, call 800-832-0034, fax 978-443-8000, or visit our website, www.jblearning.com.

Production Credits
Chairman of the Board: Clayton Jones
Chief Executive Officer: Ty Field
President: James Homer
Sr. V.P., Chief Operating Officer: Don Jones, Jr.
Sr. V.P., Chief Technology Officer: Dean Fossella
Sr. V.P., Chief Marketing Officer: Alison M. Pendergast
Sr. V.P., Chief Financial Officer: Ruth Siporin
V.P., Design and Production: Anne Spencer
V.P., Manufacturing and Inventory Control: Therese Connell
V.P., Sales, Public Safety Group: Matthew Maniscalco
Executive Publisher: Kimberly Brophy
Executive Acquisitions Editor—EMS: Christine Emerton
Associate Editor: Laura Burns

Associate Production Editor: Jessica deMartin
Director of Marketing: Alisha Weisman
Director of Sales, Public Safety Group: Patricia Einstein
Composition: diacriTech, Chennai, India
Cover Design: Kristin E. Parker
Associate Photo Researcher: Jessica Elias
Cover Image: © Mark C. Ide; background © Daniel Kvarfordt/ShutterStock, Inc.
Printing and Binding: Edwards Brothers Malloy
Cover Printing: Edwards Brothers Malloy

Editorial Credits
Author: Alan Heckman, BS, NREMT-P

ISBN: 978-1-284-04813-1

6048

Printed in the United States of America
16   10 9

Contents

EMS Systems

General Knowledge

Matching

Match each of the items in the left column to the appropriate definition in the right column.

_____ **1.** Paramedic

_____ **2.** Emergency medical technician (EMT)

_____ **3.** Advanced emergency medical technician (AEMT)

_____ **4.** Appropriate medical facility

_____ **5.** Basic life support (BLS)

_____ **6.** Advanced life support (ALS)

_____ **7.** Defibrillation

_____ **8.** Emergency medical responder (EMR)

A. Use of specialized equipment to stabilize patients

B. Emergency lifesaving procedures used to stabilize patients

C. Provides continuing care to patients transported after treatment by EMRs

D. Delivery of an electric current

E. Performs basic life support skills and limited advanced life support skills

F. Persons trained and certified to provide advanced life support

G. Trained to provide basic life support and perform other noninvasive procedures

H. The first medically trained person to arrive on the scene

Multiple Choice

Read each item carefully and then select the one best response.

_____ **1.** Medical control provided by a physician who is in contact with prehospital providers is considered:

    A. indirect.

    B. off-line.

    C. two-way.

    D. online.

_____ **2.** A physician who directs training courses, helps set medical policies, and ensures quality management of the EMS system is known as:

    A. online medical control.

    B. indirect medical control.

    C. direct medical control.

    D. unnecessary medical control.

_____ **3.** The roles and responsibilities of emergency medical responders include all of the following EXCEPT:

    A. protecting themselves.

    B. summoning appropriate assistance.

    C. performing patient assessments.

    D. directing traffic at scenes.

_____ **4.** Which of the following is not an EMR skill?

    A. Controlling airway, breathing, and circulation

    B. Treating wounds and shock

    C. Splinting injuries to stabilize extremities

    D. Cardiac monitoring

_____ **5.** The EMS system was developed to:

    A. give patients a greater chance of survival.

    B. eliminate unnecessary hospital treatment.

    C. reduce the time spent waiting for hospital treatment.

    D. make better use of physicians' time and energy.

_____ **6.** A(n) _____ is trained and certified to provide advanced life support and other medical procedures.

    A. emergency medical responder

    B. emergency medical technician

    C. paramedic

    D. ambulance attendant

_____ **7.** A BLS unit consists of:

    A. a properly equipped vehicle and EMTs.

    B. a precise measurement of blood volume.

    C. the equipment needed to treat a burn patient.

    D. a portable device for communicating with the hospital.

_____ **8.** EMS systems are evaluated by the:

    A. National Highway Traffic Safety Administration.

    B. American Academy of Orthopaedic Surgeons.

    C. American Red Cross.

    D. state agencies designated by each state.

_____ **9.** Evaluation of an EMS system includes evaluation of all of the following EXCEPT:

    A. public information and education programs.

    B. transportation systems and equipment.

    C. fatality rates.

    D. medical direction.

_____ **10.** The need for transport (as opposed to rapid or prompt transport) means that:

    A. the patient's condition requires care by medical professionals.

    B. speed of transport is of great importance.

    C. the patient's life is in danger.

    D. specialized medical attention is needed.

_____ **11.** Prompt transport to an appropriate medical facility means that the:

    A. injury is not life threatening.

    B. patient's condition is stable.

    C. patient's condition may worsen without treatment.

    D. patient is unconscious.

_____ **12.** Rapid transport to an appropriate medical facility means that:

    A. EMS personnel cannot give adequate care in the field.

    B. traffic patterns are prohibiting transport of the patient.

    C. the patient's condition is stable.

    D. the patient has requested a facility by name.

_____ **13.** Which is not a responsibility of EMRs?
   A. To gain access to the patient
   B. To seek help from bystanders
   C. To protect themselves
   D. To notify the patient's family

_____ **14.** When EMTs or paramedics arrive, the EMR should:
   A. leave the scene as quickly as possible.
   B. get statements from bystanders.
   C. assist the EMTs or paramedics.
   D. all of the above.

_____ **15.** All of the following needs to be documented by the EMR EXCEPT:
   A. condition of the patient when found.
   B. vital signs.
   C. agency and personnel who took over treatment.
   D. the color of clothing worn by the patient.

_____ **16.** Direct (online) medical control:
   A. can be accessed by an 800 number.
   B. gives information regarding a physician's training and certification.
   C. is usually done by two-way radio or wireless telephone.
   D. helps to eliminate negligence lawsuits.

_____ **17.** EMRs are a critical component of an EMS system because they are:
   A. trained in traffic control.
   B. responsible for reporting emergencies.
   C. the first medically trained personnel to arrive on the scene.
   D. able to provide both basic and advanced life support.

_____ **18.** _____ is the process by which a person, institution, or program is evaluated and recognized as meeting certain standards to ensure safe and ethical patient care.
   A. Licensure
   B. Certification
   C. Accreditation
   D. Registration

_____ **19.** Confidential medical information may be discussed with:
   A. family members.
   B. bystanders at the scene.
   C. medical personnel involved in the care of the patient.
   D. all of the above.

_____ **20.** Which of the following is _not_ a goal of EMR training?
   A. Know what you should not do.
   B. Know how to use your EMR life support kit.
   C. Know how to improvise.
   D. Know how to perform advanced skills.

_____ **21.** Ambulances were first used during:
   A. World War II.
   B. World War I.
   C. the Civil War.
   D. the Revolutionary War.

_____ **22.** What agency established the first national standard curriculum to train EMS providers?
   A. Department of Health and Human Services
   B. Department of Transportation
   C. Surgeon General's Office
   D. Department of Education

_____ **23.** Which of the following is not a responsibility of the public health department?
   A. Monitoring sanitation in restaurants
   B. Conducting immunization programs
   C. Inspecting animals for diseases
   D. Determining the incidence of contagious diseases

True/False

If you believe the statement to be more true than false, write the letter "T" in the space provided. If you believe the statement to be more false than true, write the letter "F."

_____ **1.** EMRs can sometimes play a critical role in life-or-death situations.

_____ **2.** Once EMTs or paramedics arrive on the scene, an EMR's role in an emergency situation is over.

_____ **3.** Bandaging and dressing equipment should be included in an EMR life support kit.

_____ **4.** An EMR's actions can prevent a minor situation from becoming serious.

_____ **5.** Reporting and dispatch procedures are the same in every community.

_____ **6.** EMTs are more highly trained than paramedics.

_____ **7.** EMRs should provide emergency medical care to patients even if more highly trained medical personnel are on the way.

_____ **8.** The overall leader of the EMS system is the physician or medical director.

_____ **9.** As long as you provide adequate medical care, your behavior and appearance are of little importance.

_____ **10.** In cases where large numbers of people are injured, physicians may respond to the scene of the incident.

_____ **11.** Patient care should be based on the patient's socioeconomic status and cultural background.

_____ **12.** The first medically trained person present at the scene of sudden illness or injury is called an EMT.

_____ **13.** A well-prepared EMR will have all emergency medical equipment that may possibly be needed available for use.

_____ **14.** Everyday articles found at the scene should never be used in treatment because of the danger of contamination and the spread of infectious disease.

_____ **15.** The report of an emergency incident is the first step in the EMS system.

_____ **16.** The enhanced 9-1-1 system is not considered part of the emergency services dispatch center.

_____ **17.** Fire fighters and/or law enforcement personnel should not be dispatched to a medical emergency.

_____ **18.** In a well-managed community, EMTs and paramedics will outnumber fire fighters and law enforcement officials.

_____ **19.** EMRs are responsible for determining hazards at the scene of an emergency.

_____ **20.** Documentation serves as a legal record of your treatment and may be required in the event of a lawsuit.

Crossword Puzzle

Use the clues in the column to complete the crossword puzzle.

Across

3. An emergency medical _____ is the first medically trained person to arrive on the scene.

5. Emergency lifesaving procedures performed without advanced emergency procedures to stabilize the conditions of patients who have experienced sudden illness or injury.

6. An appropriate _____ is a hospital with adequate medical resources to provide continuing care to sick or injured patients who are transported after field treatment by EMRs.

8. An emergency medical _____ is a person who is trained and certified to provide basic life support and certain other noninvasive prehospital medical procedures.

Down

1. Persons trained and certified to provide advanced life support.

2. Delivery of an electric current through a person's chest wall and heart for the purpose of ending lethal heart rhythms such as ventricular fibrillation.

4. A fire, police, or EMS agency; a 9-1-1 center; or a seven-digit telephone number used by one or all of the emergency agencies to receive and dispatch requests for emergency care.

7. A person who is able to perform basic life support skills and limited advanced life support skills.

9. The use of specialized equipment such as cardiac monitors, defibrillators, intravenous fluids, drug infusion, and endotracheal intubation to stabilize a patient's condition.

Critical Thinking

Fill-in-the-Blank

Read each item carefully and then complete the statement by filling in the missing words.

1. When you arrive at the emergency scene, park your vehicle so that it does not create a(n) _____ _____.

2. Medical information about a patient is _____ and should be shared only with other medical personnel who are involved in the care of that patient.

3. The four basic goals of EMR training are to know what not to do, know how to use the EMR life support kit, know how to _____, and know how to _____ other EMS providers.

4. Fire fighters or _____ _____ personnel are likely to be the first responders in most emergencies.

5. A(n) _____ _____ _____ _____ or _____ _____ _____ _____ usually receives the telephone call reporting an incident.

Short Answer
Complete this section with short written answers using the space provided.

1. What are the 10 standard components of an EMS system?

   _____

   _____

2. What are the three points of patient contact with the EMS system?

   _____

   _____

3. Name three things that should be included in proper documentation.

   _____

   _____

4. What are the four major goals of EMR training?

   _____

   _____

5. Why is it important to have medical oversight?

   _____

   _____

6. Name any five items that should be included in an emergency medical responder life support kit.

   _____

   _____

7. List the six components of quality improvement identified by the Institute of Medicine.

   _____

   _____

You Make the Call

The following scenario provides an opportunity to explore the concerns associated with patient management. Read the scenario and answer the question to the best of your ability.

1. You are dispatched to an emergency scene and gain access to the patient. You complete the primary assessment and stabilize the patient, then paramedics arrive on the scene to assist. What should you do?

_____

_____

_____

Workforce Safety and Wellness

General Knowledge

Matching

Match each of the items in the left column to the appropriate definition in the right column.

_____ **1.** Denial

_____ **2.** Standard precautions

_____ **3.** Bargaining

_____ **4.** Pathogens

_____ **5.** Acceptance

_____ **6.** Depression

_____ **7.** Anger

A. Recognition of the finality of the grief-causing event

B. "Why me?"

C. Trying to make a deal to postpone death and dying

D. Disbelief or rejection

E. Characterized by sadness or despair

F. Microorganisms that are capable of causing disease

G. Treat all bodily fluids as potentially infectious

Multiple Choice

Read each item carefully and then select the one best response.

_____ **1.** Techniques that can be used to prevent stress include all of the following EXCEPT:

    A. drinking an adequate amount of healthy fluids.

    B. eating a well-balanced diet.

    C. focusing on stressful events and what should have been done differently.

    D. trying to create a stress-reducing environment away from work.

_____ **2.** Hepatitis B:

    A. is a disease that is easily treated.

    B. poses no risk to the EMR.

    C. cannot be prevented.

    D. is spread by direct contact with infected blood.

_____ **3.** Critical incident stress debriefings (CISDs) are usually held:

    A. during an incident.

    B. 10 to 20 days after an incident.

    C. 24 to 72 hours after an incident.

    D. because they are mandatory.

_____ **4.** Which of the following is true of tuberculosis?

    A. It is spread by blood-to-blood contact.

    B. There are drug-resistant strains.

    C. Health care workers face a low risk of exposure.

    D. Skin tests should be performed every month.

_____ **5.** The stage of the grieving process in which the finality of death is recognized is called:

    A. depression.

    B. comprehension.

    C. conclusion.

    D. acceptance.

_____ **6.** Which of the following is not a sign of stress?

    A. Difficulty sleeping

    B. Increased efficiency

    C. Loss of appetite

    D. Inability to concentrate

_____ **7.** The first step in managing stress is to:

    A. get more sleep.

    B. recognize the signs and symptoms.

    C. change jobs.

    D. change eating habits.

_____ **8.** When you feel angry about an emergency situation that you have experienced and you discuss your anger with others, you are:

    A. showing that you are not capable.

    B. breaking the confidentiality laws.

    C. causing additional stress for others.

    D. avoiding unhealthy physical symptoms caused by bottling up your emotions.

_____ **9.** The stage of the grieving process that involves trying to negotiate a postponement of death is called:

    A. bargaining.

    B. acceptance.

    C. contracts.

    D. denial.

_____ **10.** Which of the following statements about depression is false?

    A. It is characterized by quiet or silent behavior.

    B. It is a natural reaction to a major threat or loss.

    C. Continued depression typically does not require help.

    D. It is characterized by feelings of sadness and despair.

_____ **11.** In the grieving process, a normal reaction is one of disbelief, which protects those who are experiencing the situation. This stage is called:

    A. preservation.

    B. denial.

    C. depression.

    D. skepticism.

_____ **12.** HIV stands for:

    A. human immunization virus.

    B. histamine immune vaccine.

    C. hyperinspiration vaporization.

    D. human immunodeficiency virus.

_____ **13.** Two examples of bloodborne pathogens are:

    A. HIV and hepatitis B virus.

    B. AIDS and RSI.

    C. HEPA and hepatitis B virus.

    D. PASG and CISD.

_____ **14.** HIV is transmitted by direct contact with infected:

    A. blood or semen.

    B. blood or vomitus.

    C. semen or sputum.

    D. saliva or tears.

_____ **15.** Tuberculosis is spread by contact with contaminated:

    A. blood.

    B. feces.

    C. air.

    D. all of the above.

_____ **16.** Standard precautions give guidelines for safe procedures for:

    A. transporting patients.

    B. sexual relations.

    C. responding to major natural disasters.

    D. minimizing the spread of pathogens.

_____ **17.** The standard precautions recommended by the Centers for Disease Control and Prevention (CDC) call for the use of:

    A. equipment with the OSHA seal.

    B. reflective vests and hard hats or helmets.

    C. supplies manufactured in the United States.

    D. medical gloves, protective eyewear, a face shield or mask, and handwashing.

_____ **18.** An emergency medical care provider should have:

    A. a hepatitis B vaccine.

    B. tetanus prophylaxis.

    C. a tuberculin skin test.

    D. all of the above.

_____ **19.** The most important consideration at the scene of an accident is to:

    A. make sure the scene is safe for you and others around the scene.

    B. make sure your vehicle is visible.

    C. park your vehicle as close as possible to victims.

    D. have your vehicle facing the flow of traffic.

_____ **20.** Hazardous materials situations that require special attention may occur:

    A. with vehicles marked with specific placards.

    B. in homes.

    C. at industrial sites.

    D. all of the above.

_____ **21.** Safety begins when you:

    A. encounter a violent situation.

    B. begin treatment.

    C. arrive at the scene.

    D. are dispatched to the scene.

_____ **22.** Which of the following is a not a typical hazard encountered by EMRs?

    A. Traffic

    B. Blunt objects

    C. Violence

    D. Animals

_____ **23.** Which of the following statements regarding crowds is false?

    A. You should request help from law enforcement before the crowd gets out of control.

    B. Friendly crowds do not interfere with your duties.

    C. Unfriendly crowds may require police presence.

    D. You should assess the feeling of the crowd before you get in a position from which there is no exit.

_____ **24.** If you believe that a crash involves hazardous materials:

    A. obtain a sample of the material for identification.

    B. enter the scene once you have identified the material.

    C. extricate all victims from the vehicle as quickly as possible.

    D. stop uphill and upwind and determine if the vehicle is marked with a placard.

_____ **25.** All the following statements regarding fire hazards are true EXCEPT:

    A. never enter a burning building without proper turnout gear and SCBA.

    B. keep all ignition sources away from spilled fluids.

    C. vehicles involved in a collision rarely present a fire hazard.

    D. do not exceed the limits of your training when dealing with fire.

True/False

If you believe the statement to be more true than false, write the letter "T" in the space provided. If you believe the statement to be more false than true, write the letter "F."

_____ **1.** Providing emergency medical care as an EMR is stressful only if you are unsure of what you are doing.

_____ **2.** Stress can be eliminated if you learn proper techniques.

_____ **3.** A healthy, well-balanced diet contributes to the prevention and reduction of stress.

_____ **4.** You should use CISD personnel only when you can no longer cope with your stress.

_____ **5.** Caffeine is a drug that causes an increase in blood pressure and an increase in your stress level.

_____ **6.** Alcoholic beverages should only be consumed in moderation because they reduce your ability to deal with stress.

_____ **7.** EMRs working rotating shifts or 24-hour shifts may experience disruption of normal sleep patterns.

_____ **8.** Gowns and aprons should be worn on all EMR calls.

_____ **9.** Medical gloves are adequate protection for EMRs, and there is little need to wash hands if they are worn.

_____ **10.** There is substantial evidence that HIV can be spread by direct contact with a patient's saliva or urine.

_____ **11.** You should never enter an emergency situation that is unsafe unless you have the proper training and equipment.

_____ **12.** If a person has adequate training and is competent, the services of a mental health care professional will not be needed.

_____ **13.** A health care worker in an emergency situation should decide by visual examination whether or not protective equipment for bloodborne pathogens is necessary.

_____ **14.** Receiving the hepatitis B vaccine may help to protect you against hepatitis B.

_____ **15.** Testing for the presence of tuberculosis is not recommended for EMRs unless there is a family history of the disease.

_____ **16.** To minimize exposure to tuberculosis, an EMR should use a HEPA respirator, oxygen mask, or face mask.

_____ **17.** A health care worker should assume that all patients are potential carriers of bloodborne pathogens.

_____ **18.** A used hypodermic needle needs to be cut or bent to ensure that it will not be reused.

_____ **19.** At the scene of a crime, your responsibilities are only medical in nature and do not involve any responsibility for criminal evidence.

_____ **20.** There are situations in which the EMR should wait for law enforcement personnel before approaching the scene.

_____ **21.** Service dogs are generally not possessive of their owners.

_____ **22.** Animals may present hazards such as bites, kicking, or even trampling.

_____ **23.** Methicillin-resistant *Staphylococcus aureus* (MRSA) may show up as a skin sore.

_____ **24.** Most MRSA infections occur in daycare centers and schools.

_____ **25.** EMS providers should be immunized against influenza, tetanus, and hepatitis B virus.

_____ **26.** Influenza, whooping cough, and SARS are spread by direct contact with others.

Crossword Puzzle

Use the clues in the column to complete the crossword puzzle.

Across

4. The fifth stage of the grief process, when the person experiencing grief recognizes the finality of the grief-causing event.

5. The fourth stage of the grief reaction, when the person expresses despair (an absence of cheerfulness and hope) as a result of the grief-causing event.

8. The second stage of the grief process, when the person experiencing grief becomes upset or angry at the grief-causing event or other situations.

9. A system of psychological support designed to reduce stress on emergency personnel after a major stress-producing incident.

10. The third stage of the grief reaction, when the person experiencing grief barters to change the grief-causing event.

Down

1. Preincident _____ is training about stress and stress reactions conducted for public safety personnel before they are exposed to stressful situations.

2. Microorganisms that are capable of causing disease.

3. On-scene _____ occurs when stress counselors at the scene of stressful incidents help to deal with stress reduction.

6. _____ precautions are an infection control concept that treats all body fluids as potentially infectious.

7. The first stage of a grief reaction, when the person experiencing grief rejects the grief-causing event.

Critical Thinking

Fill-in-the-Blank

Read each item carefully and then complete the statement by filling in the missing words.

1. Stress management consists of recognizing, preventing, and _____ stress.

2. Scientific studies show that most people need about _____ hours of uninterrupted sleep per night.

3. _____ stress education provides information about the stresses that you will encounter and the reactions you may experience.

4. On-scene _____ support and disaster support services provide aid on the scenes of especially stressful incidents.

5. A(n) _____ _____ _____ _____ is used to alleviate the stress reactions caused by high-stress emergency situations.

6. _____ _____ are a major cause of death and disability in law enforcement officials, fire fighters, and EMS providers.

7. _____ objects may include vehicles, trees, poles, buildings, cliffs, and piles of materials.

8. Because electricity is _____, make sure that the electrical _____ has been turned off by a(n) _____ person.

9. Latex and nitrile medical gloves can help prevent the spread of disease from blood contamination, but they provide no protection against _____ _____.

10. Weather cannot be _____ or _____.

Short Answer
Complete this section with short written answers using the space provided.

1. List three types of calls that can create a high level of stress.

_____

_____

2. List five signs or symptoms of stress.

_____

_____

3. Describe the five standard precautions recommended by the CDC.

_____

_____

4. List three things you should keep in mind when parking your vehicle at an emergency scene.

_____

_____

5. What five special rescue situations require special safety considerations, training, or equipment?

_____

_____

6. List five hazards that may be present at an accident scene and need to be considered by the EMR.

_____

_____

7. Name the five stages of the grieving process.

_____

_____

_____

You Make the Call

The following scenarios provide an opportunity to explore the concerns associated with patient management. Read the scenarios and answer the questions to the best of your ability.

1. At 4:00 AM, you are dispatched to a shooting at a residence. As you approach, two police cars leave the scene of the crime with their lights and sirens on, and dispatch informs you that law enforcement personnel believe the shooter has left the scene. What should you do?

_____

_____

_____

2. You respond to a call for a "sick person" at an apartment complex known for violence and frequent drug overdoses. When you arrive, you find a 35-year-old man standing in the doorway of his apartment. The patient is pale with sweaty skin. He tells you that he has been feeling ill for several days. He complains of night sweats, weight loss, and coughing up blood-streaked sputum for several days. The apartment complex is rather crowded and dirty. What should you do?

_____

_____

_____

Skills

Skill Drills

Skill Drill 2-1: Proper Removal of Medical Gloves

Test your knowledge of this skill by placing the photos below in the correct order. Number the first step with a "1," the second step with a "2," etc.

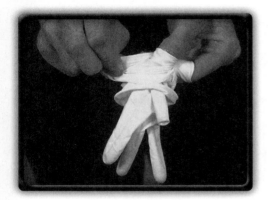

_____ Grasp both gloves with your free hand, touching only the clean interior surfaces, and gently remove the gloves.

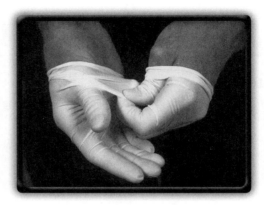

_____ Remove the second glove by pinching the exterior with the partially gloved hand.

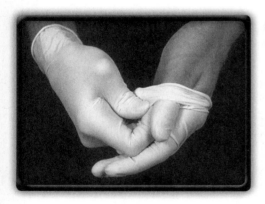

_____ Partially remove the first glove by pinching at the wrist. Be careful to touch only the outside of the glove.

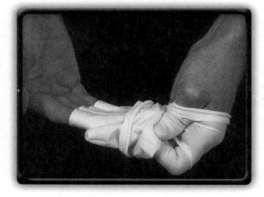

_____ Pull the second glove inside out toward the fingertips.

Medical, Legal, and Ethical Issues

General Knowledge

Matching

Match each of the items in the left column to the appropriate definition in the right column.

_____ **1.** Expressed consent

_____ **2.** Implied consent

_____ **3.** Abandonment

_____ **4.** Competent

_____ **5.** Negligence

_____ **6.** Standard of care

_____ **7.** Dependent lividity

_____ **8.** Duty to act

_____ **9.** Living will

_____ **10.** Do-not-resuscitate (DNR) order

A. EMR's legal responsibility to respond to an emergency scene and provide medical care

B. Type of consent when a patient is unconscious or when a serious threat to life exists

C. Deviation from the accepted standard of care resulting in further injury to the patient

D. Permission for treatment, given to the EMR by the patient

E. Written request giving permission to medical providers not to attempt resuscitation in the event of cardiac arrest

F. Failure of the EMR to continue emergency treatment until relieved by someone of equal or higher training

G. Legal document that states the types of medical care a person wants or does not want if they are unable to make their own treatment decisions

H. Able to make rational decisions about personal well-being

I. Blood settling to the lowest point of the body after death

J. Manner in which an individual must act or behave when giving care

Multiple Choice

Read each item carefully and then select the one best response.

_____ **1.** At the crime scene, your first priority should be to:

A. avoid touching anything that could be used as evidence.

B. provide patient care as long as your own safety is not at risk.

C. ask the patient for information about the crime.

D. make sure no witnesses leave the scene.

_____ **2.** Which of the following patients is NOT considered a minor?

A. 9-year-old girl with a broken leg

B. 12-year-old girl who is unconscious

C. 20-year-old man with a broken nose

D. 6-year-old boy with abdominal pain

_____ **3.** For negligence to occur, four conditions must be present, including all of the following EXCEPT:

A. duty to act.

B. breach of duty.

C. proximate cause.

D. death of the patient.

_____   **4.** Abandonment occurs when:

      A. patient care is terminated before another EMR or more highly trained person assumes care.

      B. you turn over patient care to a paramedic.

      C. you turn the patient over to another EMR.

      D. the patient refuses treatment by an EMR.

_____   **5.** To comply with the standard of care, you must:

      A. treat the patient to the best of your ability.

      B. provide care that a reasonable, prudent person with similar training would provide under similar circumstances.

      C. know what the local standards of care are and what statutes pertain to your community.

      D. all of the above.

_____   **6.** As an EMR, you are responsible for all the following EXCEPT:

      A. staying up to date on skills.

      B. evaluating your response times.

      C. providing care that is out of your scope.

      D. reviewing your performance.

_____   **7.** Dependent lividity:

      A. is the red or purple color that occurs on parts of the body several hours after death.

      B. is typically associated with an assault, especially in a small child or infant.

      C. occurs on the parts of the patient's body that are away from the ground.

      D. all of the above.

_____   **8.** Rigor mortis:

      A. is a sign that you should begin CPR.

      B. occurs immediately after death.

      C. is an indication that the patient cannot be resuscitated.

      D. refers to the head being separated from the body.

_____   **9.** As an EMR on the scene of an emergency, the first legal principle you need to consider is:

      A. the confidentiality of patient information.

      B. obtaining consent for treatment.

      C. whether your training qualifies you to give treatment.

      D. your duty to act.

_____   **10.** Responsibilities that concern an EMR include:

      A. professional standards of conduct.

      B. honesty.

      C. competence.

      D. all of the above.

_____   **11.** If you have made a mistake on your report, you should:

      A. try to cover it up.

      B. not put anything in writing.

      C. document the incident and not cover it up.

      D. file a claim with an attorney.

_____   **12.** Consent means:

      A. approval or permission.

      B. ethical responsibility.

      C. to confine or restrict movement.

      D. a soft-tissue injury.

_____ **13.** If a patient understands who you are and agrees to treatment, this is called:
    A. expressed consent.
    B. implied consent.
    C. assumed consent.
    D. durable power.

_____ **14.** A patient who does not refuse emergency care can be treated under the principle of:
    A. expressed consent.
    B. implied consent.
    C. protective custody.
    D. durable power.

_____ **15.** Minors:
    A. are those who are not of legal age as designated by the state.
    B. are considered to be incapable of speaking for themselves with regard to medical decisions.
    C. can be given emergency medical treatment in the field without expressed consent.
    D. all of the above.

_____ **16.** If a patient is a danger to self or to others and refuses help, an EMR may:
    A. consider calling for help from law enforcement agencies.
    B. conduct field testing to determine mental condition.
    C. leave the scene.
    D. forcefully transport the patient to the nearest appropriate treatment facility.

_____ **17.** An EMR must honor refusal of treatment if the patient:
    A. is competent.
    B. has an order of protective custody.
    C. is incompetent.
    D. is a minor.

_____ **18.** A legal document with specific instructions that state what the patient wants or does not want in terms of medical care is known as:
    A. protective custody.
    B. a living will.
    C. abandonment.
    D. durable power of attorney for health care.

_____ **19.** Which organization defines the scope of skills taught in an EMR course?
    A. HIPAA
    B. NHTSA
    C. USDOT
    D. State EMS act

_____ **20.** The failure of the EMR to continue emergency medical treatment until another qualified person assumes care is called:
    A. advance directive.
    B. incompetency.
    C. abandonment.
    D. dependent lividity.

_____ **21.** Incidents such as knife wounds, gunshot wounds, child abuse, rape, and certain infectious diseases are considered to be:

    A. reportable events.

    B. areas you are not allowed to treat.

    C. reportable only when the patient wants to press charges.

    D. not covered by Good Samaritan laws.

_____ **22.** Deviation from the accepted standard of care resulting in further injury to the patient is known as:

    A. redirection.

    B. improvisation.

    C. abandonment.

    D. negligence.

_____ **23.** Which is not a condition of negligence?

    A. Duty to act

    B. Breach of duty

    C. Resulting injuries

    D. Advance directive

_____ **24.** Most personal health information is protected under what law?

    A. NHTSA

    B. State EMS act

    C. HIPAA

    D. Advance directives

_____ **25.** Laws that protect citizens from liability for errors or omissions in giving good faith emergency care are referred to as:

    A. HIPAA.

    B. Good Samaritan laws.

    C. EMS regulations.

    D. advance directives.

True/False

If you believe the statement to be more true than false, write the letter "T" in the space provided. If you believe the statement to be more false than true, write the letter "F."

_____ **1.** To comply with the standard of care, you must treat the patient to the best of your ability.

_____ **2.** As an EMR, it is principally the responsibility of your state or agency to make sure that you maintain up-to-date skills.

_____ **3.** You have a legal duty to provide emergency care as an EMR if your agency dispatches you to a scene.

_____ **4.** Good Samaritan laws were designed to protect emergency responders from liability for errors or omissions in giving good faith care.

_____ **5.** Even if a patient is unable to communicate, the principles of law do not assume consent for treatment.

_____ **6.** EMRs should provide emergency medical care to minors even if parents or guardians are not at the scene to give permission.

_____ **7.** In some states, Good Samaritan laws do not apply to EMRs.

_____ **8.** Documentation should not include any unusual details regarding the case if they do not relate to the patient's condition or the treatment provided.

_____ **9.** Expectations concerning the standard of care may be different in different communities, cities, or counties.

_____ **10.** If a patient is not conscious, permission for treatment needs to be obtained from a family member.

_____ **11.** A rational adult can legally refuse treatment.

_____ **12.** An EMR must determine whether a living will is legally valid before beginning lifesaving procedures.

_____ **13.** Some information about a patient's care may be classified as public information.

_____ **14.** Dog bites are classified as a reportable crime.

_____ **15.** At a crime scene, a patient cannot be moved until law enforcement officials have arrived and approved movement.

Crossword Puzzle

Use the clues in the column to complete the crossword puzzle.

Across

1. _____ of attorney for health care is a legal document that allows a patient to designate another person to make medical decisions for them if they are unable to make decisions for themselves.

3. Consent actually given by a person authorizing the emergency medical responder to provide care or transportation.

6. A written request giving permission to medical personnel not to attempt resuscitation in the event of cardiac arrest.

8. Failure of the emergency medical responder to continue emergency medical treatment until relieved by someone with the same or higher level of training as the EMR.

9. A legal document that indicates what a person wants done if they cannot make their own medical decisions. Can include living wills and durable power of attorney for health care.

10. Deviation from the accepted standard of care resulting in further injury to the patient.

Down

1. Blood settling to the lowest point of the body after death, causing discoloration of the skin.

2. An emergency medical responder's legal responsibility to respond promptly to an emergency scene and provide medical care (within the limits of training and available equipment).

4. _____ laws encourage individuals to voluntarily help an injured or suddenly ill person by minimizing the liability for any errors or omissions in rendering good faith emergency care.

5. A legal document that states the types of medical care a person wants or wants withheld if they are unable to make their own treatment decisions. Sometimes called a do not resuscitate (DNR) order.

7. Able to make rational decisions about personal well-being.

Critical Thinking

Fill-in-the-Blank

Read each item carefully and then complete the statement by filling in the missing words.

1. A(n) _____ _____ is a written legal document giving specific instructions that the patient does not want to be resuscitated or kept alive by mechanical support systems.

2. Injuries caused by improper care can be found to be a situation of _____.

3. For the Good Samaritan law to provide any protection from civil liability, you must act in _____ _____ to provide care to the level of your training and to the best of your ability.

4. One who is able to make rational decisions about personal well-being is said to be _____.

5. _____ consent is based on the assumption that the patient has the right to determine what will be done to his or her body.

6. A(n) _____ is a person who has not reached legal age designated by a particular state.

7. A(n) _____ _____ _____ _____ for health care allows a patient to designate another person to make decisions about medical care for the patient if he or she is unable to make decisions for himself or herself.

8. _____ is the acronym for the Health Insurance Portability and Accountability Act of 1996.

9. Most personal health information is _____ and should not be released without the patient's permission.

10. Documentation should be clear, concise, _____, and _____.

Short Answer

Complete this section with short written answers using the space provided.

1. Which agency developed the educational standards for EMRs?

   _____

   _____

2. What is the purpose of Good Samaritan laws?

   _____

   _____

3. What four conditions can be used to reliably determine that a patient is dead?

   _____

   _____

4. Name three crimes that are reportable.

_____

_____

5. Name three factors that should be included in documentation.

_____

_____

You Make the Call

The following scenarios provide an opportunity to explore the concerns associated with patient management. Read the scenarios and answer the questions to the best of your ability.

1. You are called to the scene of a fight in a bar where a patron reportedly has been stabbed, and you consider it a potential crime scene. What should you do?

_____

_____

_____

2. You respond to a home for a "cardiac arrest." When you arrive, you are greeted by an elderly woman who is crying. The woman tells you she believes her husband is dead, and that she did not know what to do. She says she knew this day would come ever since her husband was diagnosed with terminal cancer three months ago. As you approach the patient, you notice that he is pale, unresponsive, and does not appear to be breathing. You quickly ask the woman about advance directives or a DNR. She tells you she believes something like that was done when her husband was in the hospital, but she is not sure. She asks you to do everything you can to keep him alive. What should you do?

_____

_____

_____

Communications and Documentation

CHAPTER 4

General Knowledge

Matching

Match each of the items in the left column to the appropriate definition in the right column.

_____ **1.** Base station

_____ **2.** Repeater

_____ **3.** Telemetry

_____ **4.** Mobile data terminal

_____ **5.** Paging systems

_____ **6.** Portable radio

_____ **7.** Mobile radio

_____ **8.** Fax machine

A. Hand-held, battery-operated two-way radio

B. Radio system that automatically transmits a radio signal on a different frequency

C. Process by which electronic signals are transmitted and received by radio or telephone

D. Vehicle computer terminal that sends and receives data through radio communication

E. Powerful two-way radio permanently mounted in a communications center

F. Used to send or receive printed text documents or images over a telephone or radio system

G. Communications systems used to send voice or text messages to radio receivers

H. A two-way radio that is permanently mounted in a vehicle

Multiple Choice

Read each item carefully and then select the one best response.

_____ **1.** After you have turned over the care of the patient to other EMS providers, you need to report your status to:

    A. your supervisor.

    B. your partner.

    C. the communications center.

    D. medical dispatch at the hospital.

_____ **2.** When EMTs or paramedics arrive, it is important to provide them with the:

    A. age and sex of the patient.

    B. hand-off report.

    C. complete diagnosis.

    D. care you have provided.

_____ **3.** Which one of the following is not part of the hand-off report?

    A. Postrun activity

    B. History of the incident

    C. Interventions provided

    D. Level of responsiveness

_____ **4.** In effective communication, the receiver needs to communicate that the message has been received and understood. This is called:

    A. formal communication.

    B. informal communication.

    C. nonverbal communication.

    D. feedback.

_____ 5. Do not rush when speaking to the patient. By slowing down and speaking distinctly, you can avoid:
   A. long explanations.
   B. indirect communication.
   C. having to repeat questions or explanations.
   D. writing things down.

_____ 6. Because body language is an important part of communication, you should try to avoid:
   A. kneeling next to a patient on the ground.
   B. standing relatively near to the patient.
   C. crossing your arms in front of your chest.
   D. making eye contact.

_____ 7. EMRs should speak to and treat all patients as if they were:
   A. seriously ill or injured.
   B. family members.
   C. non-English speakers.
   D. potentially dangerous.

_____ 8. Patients who are temporarily deaf will not usually:
   A. be cooperative.
   B. be able to read lips.
   C. sit still or settle down.
   D. communicate through written language.

_____ 9. If the deaf patient is with a young hearing child, resist:
   A. the urge to use the child as an interpreter.
   B. speaking to the child in front of the parent.
   C. using sign language.
   D. giving treatment with the child present.

_____ 10. Radio communications are regulated by the:
   A. FCC.
   B. NHTSA.
   C. FAA.
   D. State EMS act.

_____ 11. Which of the following is not considered effective when communicating with patients?
   A. Make eye contact with the patient.
   B. Use language the patient can understand.
   C. Speak quickly to the patient to save time.
   D. Always tell the truth.

_____ 12. Which of the following statements is false regarding communications with visually impaired patients?
   A. The patient may feel vulnerable during the chaos of the incident.
   B. It is not necessary to keep the patient and his or her service dog together.
   C. You will need to tell the patient what is happening around them.
   D. You should find out the patient's name and use it throughout your physical exam.

_____ 13. If your patient speaks a language other than English and you cannot understand each other, you should:
   A. not provide care until a certified interpreter arrives at the scene.
   B. treat the patient regardless because they will eventually understand what you are doing to them.
   C. find another way to communicate with the patient to fulfill your responsibility as an EMR to provide appropriate care.
   D. not be concerned because communication is not necessary to effectively treat patients.

_____ **14.** The medical prefix *tachy-* means:

    A. slow.

    B. heart.

    C. beyond.

    D. rapid.

_____ **15.** The medical prefix *oro-* means:

    A. denoting the nose.

    B. denoting the mouth.

    C. denoting a nerve.

    D. denoting a blood vessel.

_____ **16.** When you arrive at the scene of an incident, the first thing you should do is:

    A. begin assessing patients.

    B. request additional help.

    C. perform a visual survey of the scene.

    D. provide a verbal report to the communications center.

_____ **17.** Completing a written report and preparing your unit for the next call is part of which phase of an EMS call?

    A. Dispatch

    B. Postrun activities

    C. Arrival at the scene

    D. Update responding EMS units

True/False

If you believe the statement to be more true than false, write the letter "T" in the space provided. If you believe the statement to be more false than true, write the letter "F."

_____ **1.** In addition to radio and oral communications, EMRs must have excellent person-to-person communication skills.

_____ **2.** Along with your radio report and oral report, you must also complete a formal hand-off report for other EMS professionals at the scene.

_____ **3.** You should familiarize yourself with one communication method, such as two-way radio communications, mobile radios, or hand-held portable radios.

_____ **4.** Written documentation is important in the event of a court case because it will prevent you from being sued.

_____ **5.** Certain infectious diseases are reportable. It is important that you learn how this process is handled in your agency and what responsibilities you have in these situations.

_____ **6.** Disruptive behavior can present a danger to the patient and others and can cause delays in treatment.

_____ **7.** When dealing with young children, it is not necessary to tell them the truth about their injury or illness.

_____ **8.** If you encounter a deaf patient with whom you cannot communicate, you should rely on writing and gestures to communicate.

_____ **9.** When communicating with developmentally disabled patients, you should avoid touching the patient if touching is unnecessary.

_____ **10.** When communicating with children, you should speak in a professional manner.

_____ **11.** When you are responding to the scene of an emergency, you need to know your response area.

_____ **12.** EMRs are typically required to contact medical control to perform basic skills.

_____ **13.** Dispatch may use voice, text messaging, or an MDT to alert you to an emergency.

Crossword Puzzle

Use the clues in the column to complete the crossword puzzle.

Across

4. A process in which electronic signals are transmitted and received by radio or telephone; commonly used for sending ECG tracings.
5. A hand-held, battery-operated two-way radio.
6. Communications systems used to send voice or text messages over a radio system to specially designed radio receivers.
8. A powerful two-way radio that is permanently mounted in a communications center.

Down

1. A two-way radio that is permanently mounted in a vehicle such as a police car or fire truck.
2. A radio system that automatically retransmits a radio signal on a different frequency.
3. A device used to send or receive printed text documents or images over a telephone or radio system.
7. A computer terminal mounted in a vehicle that sends and receives data through a radio communication system.

Critical Thinking

Fill-in-the-Blank

Read each item carefully and then complete the statement by filling in the missing words.

1. A fax machine uses a(n) _____ line or _____ system to send written data.

2. A two-way radio mounted in a vehicle is a(n) _____ radio.

3. Do not assume that all older patients have _____ or _____ impairments.

4. Radio communications are regulated by the FCC, which stands for _____ _____ _____.

5. When communicating with non-English speakers, you may be able to adapt some techniques generally used to communicate with _____ patients.

6. Speak to a pediatric patient in a(n) _____ yet friendly manner.

7. _____ means excessive tension or pressure.

8. _____ is a process for verifying your actions using written records or computer-based records.

9. Cellular phones rely on _____ waves between a cellular phone and a cellular tower to propagate and receive phone messages.

10. EMTs and paramedics contact online _____ _____ to secure permission to perform certain skills.

Fill-in-the-Table

Fill in the missing parts of the table.

Prefixes Commonly Used in Medical Terminology	
Prefix	**Meaning**
Brady-	
Tachy-	
	In relation to quantities of heat
	Above, excessive, or beyond
Hypo-	
	Denoting the nose
Oro-	
Arterio-	
	Heart
Hem-, hema-, hemo-	
	Denoting nerve, nervous system, or nervous tissue
	Vessel, as in blood vessel

Short Answer

Complete this section with short written answers using the space provided.

1. What is the difference between a base station and a mobile radio?

_____

_____

2. What are the two categories of communications systems?

_____

_____

3. A portable radio is designed to be carried by rescuers. What features do these self-contained units include?

_____

_____

4. List the three types of data systems used by EMRs.

_____

_____

5. How is telemetry used by advanced life support providers?

_____

_____

6. Why is it important to introduce yourself by name and title?

_____

_____

7. Why is it important to avoid using technical medical terms when talking to a patient?

_____

_____

8. What steps should be taken when managing a patient who is exhibiting disruptive behavior?

_____

_____

You Make the Call

The following scenarios provide an opportunity to explore the concerns associated with patient management. Read the scenarios and answer the questions to the best of your ability.

1. Additional EMS personnel and paramedics arrive on the scene to care for the patient after you have completed your assessment. You need to provide them with a hand-off report. What should it include?

_____

_____

_____

2. You respond to a residence for a 32-year-old man with abdominal pain. The dispatcher informs you that this patient is deaf and that a family member will be present to help you communicate with him. What are some techniques that you can use to enhance your communication with this patient?

_____

_____

_____

The Human Body

General Knowledge

Matching

Match each of the items in the left column to the appropriate definition in the right column.

_____ **1.** Cervical spine
_____ **2.** Thoracic spine
_____ **3.** Lumbar spine
_____ **4.** Sacrum
_____ **5.** Coccyx
_____ **6.** Anterior
_____ **7.** Distal
_____ **8.** Epiglottis
_____ **9.** Superior
_____ **10.** Proximal
_____ **11.** Radius
_____ **12.** Inferior
_____ **13.** Medial
_____ **14.** Diaphragm
_____ **15.** Posterior

A. Front
B. Upper back
C. Nearer to the feet
D. Tail bone
E. Separates the chest from the abdominal cavity
F. Toward the midline
G. Lower back
H. Nearer to the free end of an extremity
I. Base of the spine
J. Describes structures closer to the trunk
K. Neck
L. Valve located at the upper end of the voice box
M. Bone located on the thumb side of the forearm
N. Back
O. Toward the head

Multiple Choice

Read each item carefully and then select the one best response.

_____ **1.** The pancreas has several functions, including the production of:
   A. bile.
   B. insulin.
   C. plasma.
   D. platelets.

_____ **2.** The removal of waste products from the body begins with which organ of the genitourinary system?
   A. Liver
   B. Urethra
   C. Kidneys
   D. Fallopian tubes

_____ **3.** The heart consists of _____ chamber(s).
   A. one
   B. two
   C. three
   D. four

_____ **4.** The bones that make up the spine are called the:

    A. ribs.

    B. xiphoid.

    C. vertebrae.

    D. sternum.

_____ **5.** The sternum is located:

    A. in the middle of the back.

    B. superior to the ribs.

    C. in the front of the chest.

    D. in the shoulder girdle.

_____ **6.** Oxygen is transported throughout the body by means of the:

    A. blood.

    B. lungs.

    C. nerves.

    D. diaphragm.

_____ **7.** Which of the following statements best describes how the circulatory system works?

    A. The heart pumps blood to the lungs to receive carbon dioxide.

    B. Blood picks up oxygen in the lungs and is then pumped by the heart to the rest of the body.

    C. Blood releases oxygen in the lungs and is then pumped by the heart back to the cells.

    D. Blood picks up oxygen in the lungs and then releases it in the heart before being pumped to the rest of the body.

_____ **8.** The large muscle that forms the bottom of the chest cavity is the:

    A. epiglottis.

    B. trachea.

    C. diaphragm.

    D. vena cava.

_____ **9.** The exchange of carbon dioxide for oxygen in the body normally occurs _____ times per minute.

    A. 8 to 10

    B. 12 to 16

    C. 18 to 22

    D. 24 to 28

_____ **10.** Which is not part of the genitourinary system?

    A. Uterus

    B. Kidneys

    C. Rectum

    D. Urethra

_____ **11.** Which is not a function of the skin?

    A. Receiving information from the outside environment

    B. Protecting the body from the environment

    C. Eliminating excess waste products

    D. Regulating body temperature

_____ **12.** All of the following are true of cardiac muscle EXCEPT:

    A. it is found only in the heart.

    B. it can live only a few minutes without an adequate supply of oxygen.

    C. it is adapted to working all the time.

    D. it can live for several hours without an adequate supply of oxygen.

_____ **13.** The brain:

    A. is part of the nervous system.

    B. may be called the body's central computer.

    C. controls the functions of thinking, voluntary actions, and involuntary functions.

    D. all of the above.

_____ **14.** Muscles that provide support and movement and are attached to bones by tendons are _____ muscles.

    A. cardiac

    B. skeletal

    C. smooth

    D. thoracic

_____ **15.** All of the following are true regarding smooth muscles EXCEPT:

    A. they are responsible for propelling food through the digestive system.

    B. they include muscles used for walking.

    C. they are part of the autonomic system.

    D. they are considered involuntary muscles.

_____ **16.** The closed, bony ring that serves as the link between the body and the lower extremities is the:

    A. femur.

    B. patella.

    C. coccyx.

    D. pelvis.

_____ **17.** The reproductive organs are protected by the:

    A. vertebrae.

    B. pelvis.

    C. intestines.

    D. xiphoid process.

_____ **18.** The longest and strongest bone in the body is the:

    A. femur.

    B. tibia.

    C. fibula.

    D. humerus.

_____ **19.** The xiphoid process is:

    A. followed at the scene of a major disaster.

    B. used to determine the competency of a patient.

    C. used when a patient is in the last stages of labor.

    D. the pointed structure at the bottom of the sternum.

_____ **20.** The rib cage:

    A. consists of 13 sets of ribs.

    B. protects the kidneys and lungs.

    C. includes the ulna and radius bones.

    D. includes the sternum, xiphoid process, and ribs.

_____ **21.** The bones of the head, collectively, are known as the:

    A. spine.

    B. skull.

    C. jaw bones.

    D. stoma.

_____ **22.** Each of the 33 bones of the spinal column is known as a:

    A. lumbar spine.

    B. sacrum.

    C. thoracic.

    D. vertebra.

_____ **23.** The tough, ropelike cords of fibrous tissue that attach muscles to bones are called:

    A. tendons.

    B. ligaments.

    C. sternum.

    D. cartilage.

_____ **24.** The fibrous bands that connect bones to bones and support and strengthen joints are called:

    A. tendons.

    B. ligaments.

    C. sternum.

    D. cartilage.

_____ **25.** The shoulder girdles consist of the:

    A. thoracic spine, clavicle, and scapula.

    B. clavicle, scapula, and humerus.

    C. vertebrae, humerus, and ulna.

    D. clavicle, humerus, and thoracic spine.

_____ **26.** Capillaries are the:

    A. lower chambers of the heart.

    B. smallest vessels in the circulatory system.

    C. small airway branches of the lungs.

    D. fluid part of the blood.

_____ **27.** Blood is returned to the heart by:

    A. veins.

    B. arteries.

    C. platelets.

    D. the aorta.

_____ **28.** Which of the following is not a function of the skeletal system?

    A. To manufacture red blood cells

    B. To protect vital structures

    C. To manufacture bile for the digestive system

    D. To support the body

_____ **29.** Blood is carried away from the heart by the:

    A. ventricles.

    B. atriums.

    C. veins.

    D. arteries.

_____ **30.** When describing a location on the body, anterior means:

    A. front.

    B. back.

    C. close.

    D. distant.

_____ **31.** When describing a location on the body, posterior means:
   A. front.
   B. back.
   C. close.
   D. distant.

_____ **32.** The term used to describe a location on the body close to the point where an arm or leg is attached is:
   A. anterior.
   B. posterior.
   C. proximal.
   D. distal.

_____ **33.** The term used to describe a location on the body that is not close to the point where an arm or leg is attached is:
   A. anterior.
   B. posterior.
   C. proximal.
   D. distal.

_____ **34.** A term to describe a body location closer to the head is:
   A. lateral.
   B. medial.
   C. superior.
   D. inferior.

_____ **35.** A term to describe a body location closer to the feet is:
   A. lateral.
   B. medial.
   C. superior.
   D. inferior.

_____ **36.** All the structures of the body that contribute to normal breathing make up which system?
   A. Respiratory
   B. Circulatory
   C. Genitourinary
   D. Digestive

_____ **37.** Which is not part of the respiratory system?
   A. Trachea
   B. Nose
   C. Kidneys
   D. Mouth

_____ **38.** Which of the following statements regarding the growth and development of infants is false?
   A. Infants can only breathe through their noses at birth.
   B. The infant's airway is very small and easily obstructed.
   C. Infants lose heat rapidly.
   D. Infants are characterized by the age group 0 to 3 years.

_____ **39.** Adolescents are characterized by what age group?
   A. 1 to 3 years
   B. 6 to 12 years
   C. 13 to 18 years
   D. 20 to 40 years

_____ **40.** The normal pulse range for an infant is:
  A. 40 to 60 beats per minute.
  B. 60 to 100 beats per minute.
  C. 100 to 160 beats per minute.
  D. 160 to 200 beats per minute.

True/False

If you believe the statement to be more true than false, write the letter "T" in the space provided. If you believe the statement to be more false than true, write the letter "F."

_____ **1.** The brain controls only voluntary actions such as speaking and moving.

_____ **2.** The spinal cord is an important part of the two-way communication system between the brain and the rest of the body.

_____ **3.** Blood is pumped away from the heart through the veins.

_____ **4.** Blood reverses the direction of its flow after delivering oxygen and nutrients to the cells.

_____ **5.** Blood cells and tissue cells exchange oxygen and carbon dioxide when the blood reaches the capillaries.

_____ **6.** A person in the standard anatomic position is standing in front of you, facing you, with hands extended over the head.

_____ **7.** Left and right, when used to describe an injury, refer to the patient's left and right.

_____ **8.** The term midline refers to an imaginary vertical line drawn from head to toe that separates the body into a left half and a right half.

_____ **9.** The term lateral refers to a wound that resembles a straight line.

_____ **10.** The term medial means closer to the midline of the body.

_____ **11.** The epiglottis helps to regulate the rate of breathing.

_____ **12.** A patient's pulse can be measured at the neck, the groin, or the wrist because of the location of veins.

_____ **13.** The upper extremity area of the skeletal system consists of the humerus, ulna, radius, wrist, and hand.

_____ **14.** Floating ribs are ribs that have been broken from the spine or sternum and are no longer attached by the ligaments.

_____ **15.** There are four different kinds of muscle.

_____ **16.** Cardiac muscle, like skeletal muscle, is found throughout the body.

_____ **17.** The skeletal and muscular systems can be considered together and called the musculoskeletal system.

_____ **18.** The organs of reproduction, together with the organs involved in the production and excretion of urine, are known as the genitourinary system.

_____ **19.** The digestive system includes the stomach, intestines, liver, rectum, bladder, and kidneys.

_____ **20.** The nervous system includes the brain, spinal cord, and individual nerves.

Labeling

Label the following diagrams with the correct terms.

1. The Respiratory System

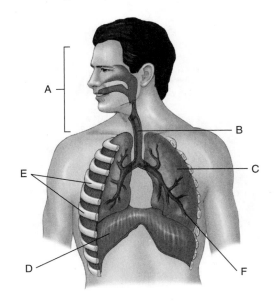

A. _____

B. _____

C. _____

D. _____

E. _____

F. _____

2. The Airway

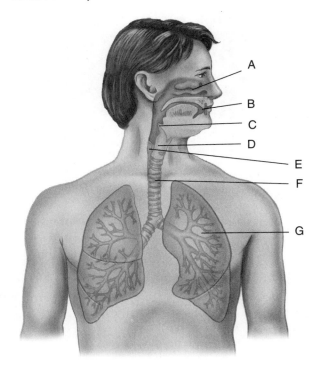

A. _____

B. _____

C. _____

D. _____

E. _____

F. _____

G. _____

3. The Circulatory System

A. _____

B. _____

C. _____

D. _____

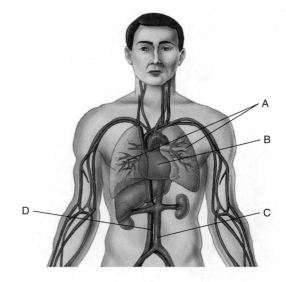

4. The Rib Cage

A. _____

B. _____

C. _____

D. _____

E. _____

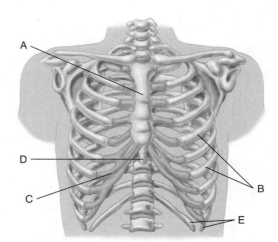

5. The Digestive System

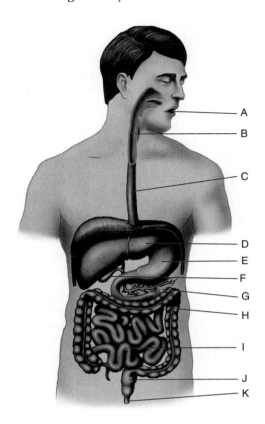

A. _____

B. _____

C. _____

D. _____

E. _____

F. _____

G. _____

H. _____

I. _____

J. _____

K. _____

Crossword Puzzle

Use the clues in the column to complete the crossword puzzle.

Across

1. The proximal portions of the upper extremity; each is made up of the clavicle, the scapula, and the humerus.
4. The breastbone.
6. A tough, elastic form of connective tissue that covers the ends of most bones to form joints; also found in some specific areas such as the nose and the ears.
7. The brain, spinal cord, and nerves.
8. Tough, ropelike cords of fibrous tissue that attach muscles to bones.
10. The 11th and 12th ribs, which do not connect to the sternum.
11. A place where two bones come into contact.
12. The 33 bones of the spinal column: 7 cervical, 12 thoracic, 5 lumbar, 5 sacral, and 4 coccygeal vertebrae.

Down

2. The upper arm bone.
3. The _____ system includes the organs of reproduction, together with the organs involved in the production and excretion of urine.
5. The fluid part of the blood that carries blood cells, transports nutrients, and removes cellular waste materials.
6. The gas formed in respiration and exhaled in breathing.
9. A hormone produced by the pancreas that enables glucose in the blood to be used by the cells of the body.

Critical Thinking

Fill-in-the-Blank

Read each item carefully and then complete the statement by filling in the missing words.

1. _____ sets of ribs protect the heart, lungs, liver, and spleen.

2. The spine is the second area of the skeletal system and consists of 33 separate bones called _____.

3. The _____ _____ is a group of nerves that carry messages to and from the brain.

4. The bones of the head include the skull and the lower _____.

5. The 11th and 12th rib sets are not attached to the sternum in any way and are called _____ ribs.

6. The lower leg has two bones, the tibia and _____.

7. Where two bones come in contact with each other, a(n) _____ is formed.

8. Cardiac muscle is found only in the _____.

9. The major organs of the digestive system are located in the _____.

10. The digestive tract begins at the _____.

Fill-in-the-Table

Fill in the missing parts of the table.

Typical Vital Sign Values Based on Age			
Age	Pulse (Heart Rate)(beats/min)	Respirations (breaths/min)	Blood Pressure (mm Hg)
Infants (newborn to age 1 year)	100-160	_____	50-95 systolic
Children (ages 1 to _____ years)	_____	15-30	80-110 systolic
Adults	60-100	12-20	_____ systolic

Short Answer

Complete this section with short written answers using the space provided.

1. Name the five parts of the airway.

   _____

   _____

2. List the three major functions of the skin.

   _____

   _____

3. Name the three major functions of the skeletal system.

   _____

   _____

4. Name the two actions of skeletal muscles that cause movement.

   _____

   _____

5. Name the five sections of the spine.

   _____

   _____

6. Name the eight parts of the digestive tract.

_____

_____

7. List the seven areas of the skeletal system.

_____

_____

You Make the Call

The following scenarios provide an opportunity to explore the concerns associated with patient management. Read the scenarios and answer the questions to the best of your ability.

1. You arrive at a scene where you are told that a 14-year-old boy has fallen about 10 feet and is lying semiconscious underneath the bleachers at a football field. You determine that you will need to check the three major pulse points. What should you do?

_____

_____

_____

2. You respond to a house fire and are directed to a 53-year-old man with burns to his chest, abdomen, and legs. You immediately assess the patient for life-threatening injuries and arrange for prompt transport. You know that this patient needs to get to a burn center as soon as possible to preserve the three major functions of the skin. What are those functions and how do they affect this patient?

_____

_____

_____

Airway Management

General Knowledge

Matching

Match each of the items in the left column to the appropriate definition in the right column.

_____ **1.** Oropharynx

_____ **2.** Trachea

_____ **3.** Alveoli

_____ **4.** Nasopharynx

_____ **5.** Aspirator

_____ **6.** Gag reflex

_____ **7.** Mandible

_____ **8.** Flowmeter

_____ **9.** Minute ventilation

_____ **10.** Stoma

_____ **11.** Pulse oximetry

_____ **12.** Bronchi

_____ **13.** Alveolar ventilation

_____ **14.** Rescue breathing

_____ **15.** Oxygen

A. Posterior part of the nose

B. Involuntary effort to vomit

C. Air pulled into and out of the lungs in 1 minute

D. Posterior part of the mouth

E. Air sacs of the lungs where the exchange of oxygen and carbon dioxide takes place

F. Controls and measures the flow of oxygen from an oxygen tank

G. Windpipe

H. Measures oxygen saturation in the capillaries

I. Lower jaw

J. Colorless, odorless gas that is essential for life

K. Suction device

L. Artificial means of breathing for a patient

M. Surgical opening that connects the windpipe to the skin

N. Exchange of oxygen and carbon dioxide in the alveoli

O. Two main branches of the windpipe

Multiple Choice

Read each item carefully and then select the one best response.

_____ **1.** The correct way to open the airway of an unconscious adult with no suspected spinal injury is to use the:

   A. head tilt–chin lift maneuver.

   B. head lift–chin tilt maneuver.

   C. head tilt–jaw lift maneuver.

   D. head lift–jaw lift maneuver.

_____ **2.** If a patient has experienced a head or neck injury, you should use the _____ maneuver to open the patient's airway.

   A. head tilt–chin lift

   B. chin thrust–jaw lift

   C. tongue–jaw lift

   D. jaw–thrust

_____ **3.** Finger sweeps:

   A. require special equipment.

   B. are performed only as a last resort.

   C. should not be performed by EMRs.

   D. should only be performed while wearing medical gloves.

_____ **4.** Mechanical suctioning of an adult should not last more than _____ seconds.
    A. 5
    B. 10
    C. 15
    D. 20

_____ **5.** Mechanical suctioning of an infant should not last more than _____ seconds.
    A. 5
    B. 10
    C. 15
    D. 20

_____ **6.** To select the proper size of a nasal airway, measure:
    A. from the bottom of the nose to the top of the ear.
    B. from the earlobe to the tip of the nose.
    C. from the bottom of the nose to the bottom of the ear.
    D. from the tip of the nose to the top of the ear.

_____ **7.** Coat the nasal airway with:
    A. petroleum-based lubricant.
    B. water.
    C. water-soluble lubricant.
    D. nothing; no lubricant is needed.

_____ **8.** If an unconscious person is lying on his or her back, the passage of air into the lungs may be blocked by the:
    A. larynx.
    B. tongue.
    C. epiglottis.
    D. relaxed diaphragm.

_____ **9.** Which of the following statements regarding the respiratory system is false?
    A. The lungs are located on either side of the heart.
    B. The lungs consist of soft, spongy tissue that contains small muscle fibers.
    C. The epiglottis prevents food or water from entering the airway.
    D. Alveoli are surrounded by capillaries.

_____ **10.** If your assessment shows that a person is not breathing but has a pulse, you should immediately:
    A. begin rescue breathing.
    B. check for signs of injury.
    C. ask bystanders for help.
    D. assume the person is dead.

_____ **11.** If a patient is breathing, you should:
    A. begin rescue breathing.
    B. begin external chest compressions.
    C. check for the odor of alcohol and, if present, let the patient sleep.
    D. check the rate and depth of the breathing and continue to maintain the airway during your assessment.

_____ **12.** When performing rescue breathing, you should remember to:
    A. blow gently enough so that the chest does not rise.
    B. pause for as little time as possible between breaths so the patient's chest does not have time to deflate.
    C. continue the head tilt–chin lift or jaw-thrust technique.
    D. blow as forcefully as possible to completely inflate all lung areas.

_____ 13. When ventilating an adult patient, each rescue breath should last for _____ second(s).

    A. 1

    B. 2

    C. $2\frac{1}{2}$

    D. 3

_____ 14. Which of the following techniques should you first use to open the airway of an unconscious infant?

    A. Jaw-thrust

    B. Finger sweep

    C. Head tilt only

    D. Head tilt–chin lift

_____ 15. The head of an infant should be tilted back only slightly, if at all, because:

    A. no pressure should be placed on the back of an infant's head.

    B. tilting the head back could block the airway.

    C. the infant's mouth and nose will close if you tilt the head too far.

    D. tilting the head back too far will place too much pressure on the forehead.

_____ 16. Another difference between infant and adult rescue breathing is that infants need:

    A. smaller, more frequent breaths.

    B. smaller, less frequent breaths.

    C. larger, more frequent breaths.

    D. larger, less frequent breaths.

_____ 17. You know you are blowing hard enough while performing rescue breathing when:

    A. the patient revives.

    B. the patient's chest rises slightly.

    C. you begin to feel lightheaded.

    D. you feel slightly out of breath.

_____ 18. You are eating in a restaurant when a woman at the next table begins coughing violently. When you ask her if she is choking, she nods and continues to cough. You should:

    A. perform the Heimlich maneuver.

    B. encourage her to cough and wait for her to become unconscious before performing the Heimlich maneuver.

    C. encourage her to cough, monitor her carefully, and arrange for transport to a hospital.

    D. demand that she answer your question out loud so you can determine whether or not her airway is completely blocked.

_____ 19. The woman suddenly stops coughing and grabs at her throat. You tell her to cough, and she shakes her head violently from side to side. You should:

    A. try to convince the woman that she should still cough.

    B. perform the Heimlich maneuver if she loses consciousness.

    C. perform the Heimlich maneuver until the object is expelled or the woman loses consciousness.

    D. alert the EMS system that rapid transport is now required.

_____ 20. In performing the Heimlich maneuver, your fist should be placed between the person's:

    A. navel and pubis.

    B. navel and xiphoid process.

    C. heart and xiphoid process.

    D. sternum and xiphoid process.

_____ **21.** If an oxygen cylinder contains less than _____, it should be replaced with a full cylinder.

    A. 500 psi

    B. 1,000 psi

    C. 1,500 psi

    D. 2,000 psi

_____ **22.** Which of the following statements regarding oxygen administration is false?

    A. A nonrebreathing mask is typically used to deliver 4 to 6 liters per minute of oxygen.

    B. A nasal cannula can deliver oxygen concentrations near 90%.

    C. High pressure in an oxygen cylinder can cause an explosion if the cylinder is damaged.

    D. The portable oxygen cylinders used by most EMS systems are either size D or E.

_____ **23.** The posterior part of the mouth used in breathing is:

    A. the oropharynx.

    B. the nasopharynx.

    C. the trachea.

    D. none of the above.

_____ **24.** The posterior part of the nose used in breathing is:

    A. the oropharynx.

    B. the nasopharynx.

    C. the trachea.

    D. all of the above.

_____ **25.** Parts of the body used in breathing include:

    A. the oropharynx and nasopharynx.

    B. the trachea and chest muscles.

    C. the lungs and diaphragm.

    D. all of the above.

_____ **26.** The air sacs of the lungs where the exchange of oxygen and carbon dioxide takes place are:

    A. bronchi.

    B. alveoli.

    C. tracheae.

    D. none of the above.

_____ **27.** The first step in assessing a patient's airway is to:

    A. place the patient on his or her back.

    B. look and listen for signs of breathing.

    C. check for responsiveness.

    D. use the head tilt–chin lift technique.

_____ **28.** A patient's airway may be cleared with:

    A. manual suction devices.

    B. finger sweeps.

    C. aspirators.

    D. all of the above.

_____ **29.** All of the following are true regarding mechanical suction devices EXCEPT:

    A. you should not suction for longer than 15 seconds with an adult.

    B. devices usually have two different tips.

    C. the suction catheter should be fed past the point of visualization to suction deeper parts of the airway.

    D. devices are either battery-powered or oxygen-powered.

_____ **30.** Which of the following is not a sign of inadequate breathing?

    A. A respiratory rate of 12 to 20 breaths per minute

    B. Pale or blue skin

    C. Rapid or gasping respirations

    D. Wheezing or gurgling

_____ **31.** Respiratory arrest can be caused by all of the following EXCEPT:

    A. poisoning.

    B. drug overdose.

    C. extremity fractures.

    D. severe loss of blood.

_____ **32.** The recovery position may help keep the airway open:

    A. if the patient has not sustained trauma.

    B. by allowing secretions to drain out of the mouth.

    C. because gravity will help keep the patient's tongue and lower jaw from blocking the airway.

    D. all of the above.

_____ **33.** An oral airway:

    A. should not be used in any unconscious patient.

    B. can serve as the pathway through which you can suction a patient.

    C. cannot be used with mechanical breathing devices.

    D. all of the above.

_____ **34.** Which of the following is true regarding rescue breathing?

    A. Rescue breaths should be provided at a rate of 10 to 12 breaths per minute for infants, children, and adults.

    B. It may involve a mouth-to-mask device or a barrier device.

    C. It requires specific equipment to be successful.

    D. It is not part of the skill set for EMRs.

_____ **35.** Mouth-to-mask rescue breathing allows the rescuer to do all of the following EXCEPT:

    A. add the use of supplemental oxygen.

    B. perform rescue breathing without mouth-to-mouth contact.

    C. reduce his or her risk of transmitting infectious diseases.

    D. protect the airway from aspiration of secretions.

_____ **36.** To perform mouth-to-mask rescue breathing:

    A. follow steps similar to those used for mouth-to-mouth rescue breathing.

    B. two rescuers are needed.

    C. the rescuer must have supplemental oxygen.

    D. all of the above.

_____ **37.** Which of the following statements regarding pulse oximetry is false?

    A. It helps to determine whether your treatment is helping the patient.

    B. It works well on people wearing nail polish.

    C. It will give you a false reading in a carbon monoxide poisoning situation.

    D. It measures light that passes through a fingertip or earlobe.

_____ **38.** When ventilating a patient with a tracheal stoma, you should:

    A. avoid hyperextending the patient's head and neck.

    B. not remove the breathing tube for any reason.

    C. always seal the mouth and nose of every patient before ventilating.

    D. not use a bag-mask device.

True/False

If you believe the statement to be more true than false, write the letter "T" in the space provided. If you believe the statement to be more false than true, write the letter "F."

_____ 1. Brain cells are the most sensitive cells in the human body.

_____ 2. If a foreign object completely blocks the airway, a patient will lose consciousness in 3 to 4 minutes.

_____ 3. If the Heimlich maneuver is successful in removing a foreign object from a person's airway, medical care is considered complete.

_____ 4. In an unconscious patient, the head tilt–chin lift or jaw-thrust techniques are effective in opening an airway obstructed by a foreign object.

_____ 5. If a person is coughing or gagging, you can assume the airway is only partially obstructed.

_____ 6. Coughing is the most effective way for a person to bring up a foreign object partially blocking the airway.

_____ 7. Air that cannot be exhaled but that remains in the lungs can pop an object out when the air is compressed by properly administered abdominal thrusts.

_____ 8. A stoma is an opening in the neck.

_____ 9. If a patient's chest rises during mouth-to-stoma breathing, you should seal the mouth and nose with one hand.

_____ 10. A stoma may have to be cleared of mucus before mouth-to-stoma breathing is begun.

_____ 11. Always insert the manual suction device just beyond where you can see.

_____ 12. Suctioning the airway is a lifesaving technique.

_____ 13. Unconscious patients will not be able to keep their airways open.

_____ 14. Usually a patient will tolerate a nasal airway better than an oral airway.

_____ 15. A normal breathing rate in an adult is 12 to 20 breaths per minute.

_____ 16. A mouth-to-mask ventilator device consists of a mask that fits the rescuer's mouth and a mouthpiece.

_____ 17. The recovery position helps to maintain an open airway in an unconscious patient.

_____ 18. The lower jaw is called the mandible.

_____ 19. Strong muscles are an important part of healthy lungs.

_____ 20. The decision to use the head tilt–chin lift technique or the jaw-thrust technique should be made after determining the type of blockage found in the patient's airway.

_____ 21. Use of the head tilt–chin lift technique on a patient who has neck injuries may cause further damage.

_____ 22. The jaw-thrust maneuver should never be attempted on a patient who may have injuries to the neck.

_____ 23. The recovery position can be used to keep the airway open once a patient is breathing adequately.

_____ 24. If an unconscious patient is breathing adequately, the airway can be kept open with the use of an oral or nasal airway.

_____ 25. Nasal airways can only be used in an unconscious patient.

_____ 26. Adequate breathing in a patient can be determined by looking, listening, and feeling.

_____ 27. Mouth-to-mouth rescue breathing puts the rescuer at a higher risk of contracting a disease.

_____ 28. In performing rescue breathing for an infant, you must extend the head back as far as possible.

_____ 29. Rescue breathing for children is done at a slightly slower rate than for adults.

_____ 30. The most common foreign object that causes airway obstruction is food.

_____ 31. If a patient can speak or cough, the airway is only partially obstructed.

_____ **32.** Oxygen can burn or explode by itself.

_____ **33.** Pulse oximetry is reliable in patients with hypothermia or severe blood loss.

_____ **34.** With sufficient training and practice, a single rescuer can ventilate a patient using a bag-mask device.

_____ **35.** A bag-mask device can deliver up to 90% oxygen to a patient if 4 to 6 liters per minute of oxygen is supplied into the reservoir bag.

Labeling

Label the following diagrams with the correct terms.

1. Airway Maintenance

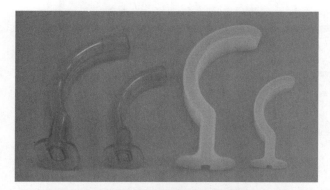

A. _____

B. _____

C. _____

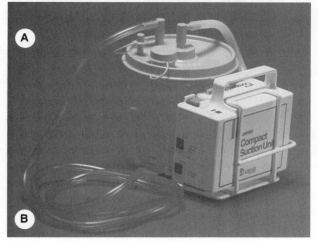

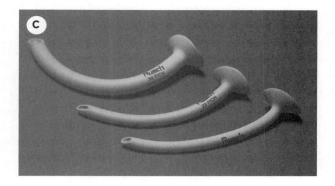

2. Assisted Ventilation

A. _____

B. _____

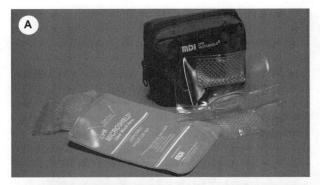

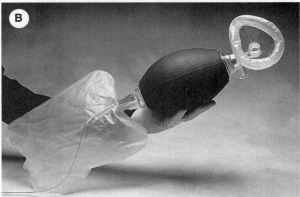

Crossword Puzzle

Use the clues in the column to complete the crossword puzzle.

Across

1. External cardiac _____ are a means of applying artificial circulation by applying rhythmic pressure and relaxation on the lower half of the sternum.

3. The passages from the openings of the mouth and nose to the air sacs in the lungs through which air enters and leaves the lungs.

7. The artificial circulation of the blood and movement of air into and out of the lungs in a pulseless, nonbreathing patient.

8. The tube through which food passes. It starts at the throat and ends at the stomach.

10. The organs that supply the body with oxygen and eliminate carbon dioxide from the blood.

11. An airway adjunct that is inserted into the nostril of a patient who is not able to maintain a natural airway. It is also called a nasopharyngeal airway.

12. A machine that consists of a monitor and a sensor probe that measures the oxygen saturation in the capillary beds.

Down

2. A mechanical breathing device used to administer mouth-to-mask rescue breathing.

4. A clear plastic tube, used to deliver oxygen, that fits onto the patient's nose.

5. A clear plastic mask used for oxygen administration that covers the mouth and nose.

6. An airway adjunct that is inserted into the mouth to keep the tongue from blocking the upper airway. It is also called an oropharyngeal airway.

9. The smallest blood vessels that connect small arteries and small veins. Capillary walls serve as the membrane to exchange oxygen and carbon dioxide.

Critical Thinking

Fill-in-the-Blank

Read each item carefully and then complete the statement by filling in the missing words.

1. Two types of suction devices are _____ and _____.

2. If a patient is breathing adequately, you can keep the airway open by placing the patient in the _____ position.

3. The major signs of respiratory arrest are no chest movement, no breath sounds, no air movement, and _____.

4. The most critical sign of inadequate breathing is _____ _____.

5. To perform rescue breathing, pinch the patient's _____ with your thumb and forefinger.

6. The patient's airway is the pipeline that transports _____ _____ from the lungs.

7. Without oxygen, the brain will die in _____ to _____ minutes.

8. In cases of severe head trauma, a(n) _____ airway may cause further brain damage.

9. Key words in caring for a patient's airway are "_____" and "_____."

10. Before insertion of an oral airway, the proper size must be determined by measuring from the patient's _____ to the corner of the _____.

Short Answer

Complete this section with short written answers using the space provided.

1. Name the two primary purposes of an oral airway.

_____

_____

2. List the steps involved in inserting an oral airway.

_____

_____

3. List the steps involved in inserting a nasal airway.

_____

_____

4. List the steps involved in ventilating a patient with a mouth-to-mask device.

_____

_____

5. Name two signs of inadequate breathing.

_____

_____

6. Name two types of airway obstructions.

_____

_____

7. Describe how to place a patient in the recovery position.

_____

_____

8. List the advantages to maintaining an airway by supporting the head and cervical spine for a patient trapped in a motor vehicle.

_____

_____

You Make the Call

The following scenarios provide an opportunity to explore the concerns associated with patient management. Read the scenarios and answer the questions to the best of your ability.

1. You are called to a scene where an unconscious 18-year-old has choked on a piece of food and has a severe airway obstruction. You treat this patient by performing CPR. What should you have done differently if this patient had been conscious when you arrived?

_____

_____

_____

2. You are dispatched to a local church for a possible cardiac arrest. When you enter the room, you find a 72-year-old man lying on the floor surrounded by people. The patient has a tracheal stoma and does not appear to be breathing adequately. A woman from the church tells you that she would have started mouth-to-mouth but was unsure of how to proceed due to the stoma. What should you do?

_____

_____

_____

Skills

Skill Drills

Skill Drill 6-2: Inserting an Oral Airway
Test your knowledge of this skill by filling in the correct words in the photo caption.

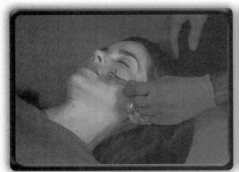 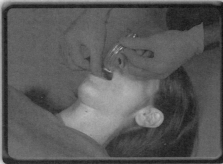 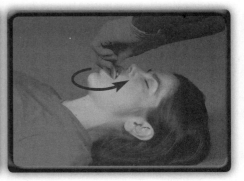

1. Size the airway by measuring from the patient's _____ to the corner of the mouth.

2. Insert the _____ _____ upside down along the roof of the patient's mouth until you feel resistance.

3. Rotate the airway _____ degrees until the flange comes to rest on the patient's lips or teeth.

Skill Drill 6-3: Inserting a Nasal Airway
Test your knowledge of this skill by filling in the correct words in the photo caption.

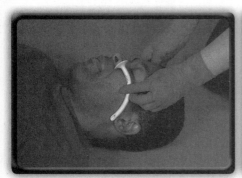 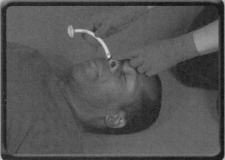 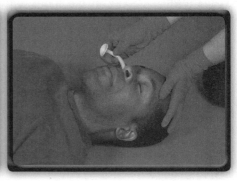

1. Size the _____ by measuring from the tip of the patient's nose to the patient's earlobe.

2. Insert the lubricated airway into the _____ nostril.

3. Advance the airway until the flange rests against the _____.

Skill Drill 6-6: Using a Bag-Mask Device With One Rescuer
Test your knowledge of this skill by filling in the correct words in the photo caption.

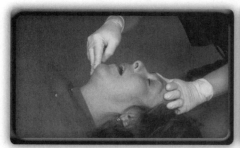

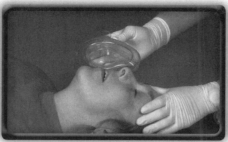

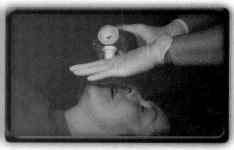

1. Kneel at the patient's _____ and maintain an open airway. Check the patient's mouth for _____, foreign bodies, and _____.

2. Select the proper _____ size.

3. Place the mask over the patient's _____.

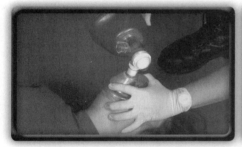

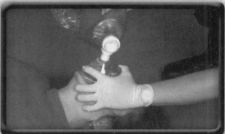

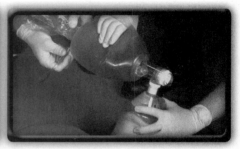

4. _____ the mask.

5. _____ the bag with your other hand. Check for chest _____.

6. Add _____ _____.

Skill Drill 6-7: Performing Infant Rescue Breathing
Test your knowledge of this skill by filling in the correct words in the photo caption.

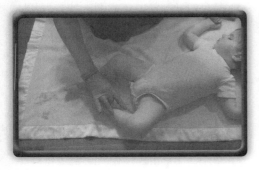

1. Establish the patient's level of
_____.

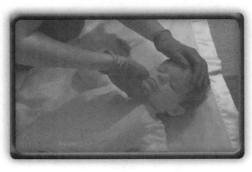

2. Open the infant's airway using
the _____
_____
_____
_____ maneuver.

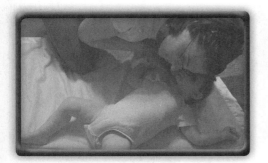

3. Check for _____.

4. Perform infant _____
breathing.

Professional Rescuer CPR

General Knowledge

Matching

Match each of the items in the left column to the appropriate definition in the right column.

_____	**1.** Brachial pulse	**A.** Movement of air into and out of the lungs
_____	**2.** Child	**B.** Thumb side of the wrist
_____	**3.** Plasma	**C.** Wave of pressure created by the heart during contractions
_____	**4.** Carotid pulse	**D.** Between 1 year of age and the onset of puberty
_____	**5.** Ventilations	**E.** Taken at the groin
_____	**6.** Pulse	**F.** Inside of the upper arm
_____	**7.** Femoral pulse	**G.** Carries blood cells, transports nutrients, and removes cellular waste
_____	**8.** Infant	**H.** Taken on either side of the neck
_____	**9.** Gastric distention	**I.** Inflation of the stomach with air from aggressive ventilations
_____	**10.** Radial pulse	**J.** Younger than 1 year of age

Multiple Choice

Read each item carefully and then select the one best response.

_____ **1.** A woman who collapses on the beach is unresponsive and is not breathing when you arrive. She has no pulse. You should:

    A. begin CPR, starting with chest compressions.

    B. interview bystanders.

    C. search her purse for identification.

    D. check her arms and legs for sting marks.

_____ **2.** Which of the following is not a component of blood?

    A. Plasma

    B. Platelets

    C. Red and white blood cells

    D. Epithelial cells

_____ **3.** What part of your hand should you place on an adult's sternum to deliver chest compressions?

    A. Thumb

    B. First three fingers

    C. Heel of the hand

    D. Back of the hand in a fisted position

_____ **4.** Signs of cardiac arrest in children are _____ those of an adult.

    A. completely different from

    B. the same as

    C. more easily observed than

    D. less easily observed than

_____ **5.** If you are alone with an adult patient who needs CPR, you should:

      A. perform CPR for 1 minute before activating the EMS system.

      B. perform CPR for 3 minutes before activating the EMS system.

      C. perform CPR for 5 minutes before activating the EMS system.

      D. activate the EMS system before beginning CPR.

_____ **6.** What is the ratio of chest compressions to ventilations in one-rescuer adult CPR?

      A. 5 to 2

      B. 10 to 2

      C. 15 to 2

      D. 30 to 2

_____ **7.** What is the ratio of chest compressions to ventilations in two-rescuer adult CPR?

      A. 5 to 2

      B. 10 to 2

      C. 15 to 2

      D. 30 to 2

_____ **8.** In one-rescuer adult CPR, each set of chest compressions should be delivered within _____ seconds.

      A. 10

      B. 15

      C. 18

      D. 30

_____ **9.** After giving chest compressions and ventilations for 2 minutes, you should:

      A. turn the patient.

      B. continue cycles of compressions and ventilations until an AED arrives or the patient moves.

      C. check the eyes.

      D. stop CPR to see if the patient has responded.

_____ **10.** You should use _____ finger(s) to deliver chest compressions to an infant.

      A. 1

      B. 2

      C. 3

      D. 4

_____ **11.** An alternative method for doing chest compressions on an infant is:

      A. three-finger compressions.

      B. two-finger/encircling hands technique.

      C. one-thumb compression technique.

      D. two-thumb/encircling hands technique.

_____ **12.** An infant's chest should be compressed:

      A. 0" to 1".

      B. 1" to 1½".

      C. 1½" to 2".

      D. at least one third the depth of the chest.

_____ **13.** A child's chest should be compressed:

      A. 0" to 1".

      B. 1" to 1½".

      C. 1½" to 2".

      D. at least one third the depth of the chest.

_____ **14.** In two-rescuer CPR, the ratio of chest compressions to ventilations for both infants and children should be:
- **A.** 5 to 1.
- **B.** 5 to 2.
- **C.** 10 to 1.
- **D.** 15 to 2.

_____ **15.** In what position should you place an infant to deliver effective CPR?
- **A.** Lying on a firm surface
- **B.** Lying on pillows
- **C.** Lying in your arms
- **D.** Upright in your arms

_____ **16.** If you hear a cracking sound as you are performing CPR, you should:
- **A.** stop CPR and wait for additional help to arrive.
- **B.** stop CPR until you can determine whether the patient's ribs are broken.
- **C.** continue CPR but check and/or adjust the position of your hands.
- **D.** continue CPR without stopping because ribs sometimes break even when CPR is performed properly.

_____ **17.** Two rescuers find an unconscious woman lying on the ground next to her automobile. There are no bystanders or other rescue personnel at the scene. It would be most appropriate for:
- **A.** one rescuer to activate the EMS system but only if the patient needs CPR.
- **B.** one rescuer to activate the EMS system while the other examines the patient and begins CPR, if necessary.
- **C.** both rescuers to perform two-rescuer CPR for several minutes and activate the EMS system only if the patient does not respond.
- **D.** both rescuers to perform two-rescuer CPR for 1 minute and then switch to one-rescuer CPR while the second rescuer activates the EMS system.

_____ **18.** What part of the heart pumps highly oxygenated blood to the rest of the body?
- **A.** Right atrium
- **B.** Left atrium
- **C.** Right ventricle
- **D.** Left ventricle

_____ **19.** Oxygen passes from the blood cells into the cells of the body via:
- **A.** veins.
- **B.** arteries.
- **C.** capillaries.
- **D.** lymphatics.

_____ **20.** When performing rescue breathing on an adult patient, each rescue breath should be given over a period of _____ second(s).
- **A.** 1
- **B.** $1^1/_2$
- **C.** 2
- **D.** 3

_____ **21.** An automated external defibrillator (AED) will do all of the following EXCEPT:
- **A.** analyze the patient's heart rhythm.
- **B.** deliver a shock to the patient.
- **C.** check the patient's pulse.
- **D.** recommend a shock.

_____ **22.** You should discontinue CPR when:
- **A.** there are reliable criteria for death.
- **B.** you are too exhausted to continue.
- **C.** a physician assumes responsibility for the patient.
- **D.** all of the above.

_____ **23.** Chest compression:

    A. mimics the squeezing and relaxation cycles of a normal heart.

    B. should be used if there is no carotid pulse.

    C. requires a firm horizontal surface.

    D. all of the above.

_____ **24.** The three parts of CPR can be remembered with the letters:

    A. SAMPLE.

    B. ABC.

    C. AVPU.

    D. DNR.

_____ **25.** Which is not a link in the American Heart Association's Chain of Survival?

    A. Early CPR

    B. Early access to EMS system

    C. Early diagnosis of cause

    D. Early advanced care by paramedics and hospital personnel

_____ **26.** Which of the following is not a sign of effective CPR?

    A. Compressions and ventilations are delivered at a slow pace.

    B. The chest visibly rises during ventilations.

    C. The carotid pulse is present during chest compression.

    D. The patient's skin color improves.

_____ **27.** If the patient regurgitates during resuscitation, you should:

    A. stop what you are doing and wait for advanced help to arrive.

    B. sit the patient up to help protect the airway.

    C. immediately turn the patient onto his or her side to allow vomitus to drain from the mouth.

    D. continue chest compressions without interruption.

_____ **28.** Cardiac arrest means that:

    A. the heart suddenly stops functioning.

    B. oxygen is not getting to the body's organs.

    C. a patient is unconscious and not breathing.

    D. all of the above.

_____ **29.** The discontinuation of CPR without the order of a physician or without turn in care over to someone of equal or higher training could be considered:

    A. neglect.

    B. abandonment.

    C. assault.

    D. battery.

_____ **30.** The heart consists of _____ chambers.

    A. two

    B. three

    C. four

    D. five

True/False

If you believe the statement to be more true than false, write the letter "T" in the space provided. If you believe the statement to be more false than true, write the letter "F."

_____   **1.** If a valid do not resuscitate (DNR) order is present, you can withhold CPR.

_____   **2.** If you are delivering chest compressions properly, your downward pushes should be smooth and rhythmic.

_____   **3.** By interlocking your fingers during chest compressions, you will avoid digging into (and potentially hurting) the patient with your fingers.

_____   **4.** To be sure you are relaxing chest compressions completely, you should lift your hand off the patient's chest after each compression.

_____   **5.** Both your fingers and a clean cloth can be used to clear a patient's mouth of vomitus.

_____   **6.** A patient should not be moved or turned simply to clear the mouth of vomitus.

_____   **7.** If a patient regurgitates while you are performing CPR, you must clear away the vomitus before resuming CPR.

_____   **8.** If a patient's heart has stopped, rescue breathing alone will not save the patient.

_____   **9.** An adult heart is about the size of a fist.

_____   **10.** Between chest compressions, the heart relaxes and refills with blood automatically.

_____   **11.** Chest compressions should be done on patients whose hearts have not yet stopped.

_____   **12.** Chest compressions should be done along with rescue breathing for oxygen to travel throughout the body.

_____   **13.** One-rescuer CPR is more effective than two-rescuer CPR.

_____   **14.** Because two-rescuer CPR is less tiring than one-rescuer CPR, rescuers are generally able to perform it for a longer period of time.

_____   **15.** The two rescuers should be on the same side of a patient during two-rescuer CPR.

_____   **16.** In two-rescuer CPR, the compressor should give the ventilator enough time to fully ventilate the patient after each 10th compression.

_____   **17.** In two-rescuer CPR, the ventilator provides the oxygen that the compressor is trying to keep circulating through the patient's body.

_____   **18.** During two-rescuer CPR, if the two rescuers have practiced together before, the compressor may count compressions silently.

_____   **19.** If a patient vomits during CPR, it is unpleasant for the rescuer, but it creates no danger to the patient.

_____   **20.** Before beginning CPR, rescuers should consider the amount of space needed to administer CPR.

_____   **21.** An EMR needs to know about any living wills or advance directives a patient may have before starting CPR.

_____   **22.** To perform chest compressions effectively, you should straddle the patient.

_____   **23.** To perform chest compressions effectively, the location of the hands in relation to the sternum is of critical importance.

_____   **24.** When performing chest compressions, improper placement of the rescuer's hands can cause damage to the patient's lungs and ribs.

_____   **25.** Chest compressions on an adult should be at the rate of 30 compressions per minute.

_____   **26.** The steps for child CPR are essentially the same as for an adult with some modifications.

_____   **27.** Chest compressions on an infant require the use of the heel of only one hand.

_____   **28.** The compression-to-breath ratio for two-rescuer CPR in a child is 30 compressions followed by 2 breaths.

_____ **29.** Chest compressions on a child may require the use of the heel of only one hand.

_____ **30.** If there are signs of dependent lividity, CPR should not be started.

_____ **31.** You should make sure that everyone is "clear" of the patient before pushing the shock button on an AED.

_____ **32.** An AED is safe to use in infants older than 1 month of age.

Labeling

Label the following diagram with the correct terms.

1. Pulse Locations

A. _____

B. _____

C. _____

D. _____

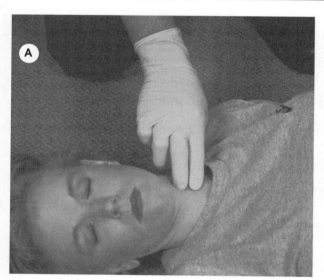

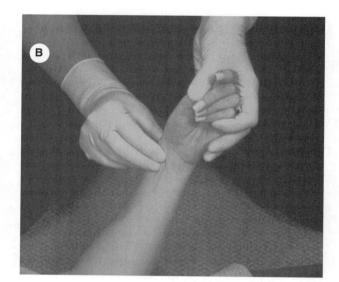

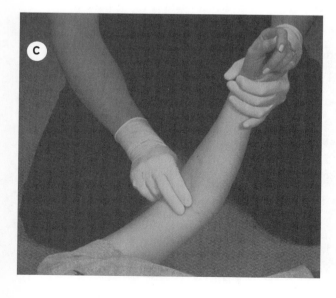

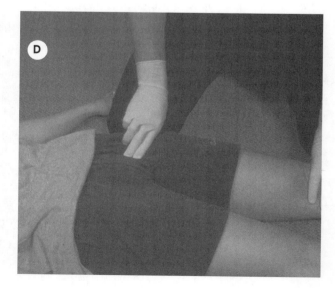

Crossword Puzzle

Use the clues in the column to complete the crossword puzzle.

Across

3. Microscopic disc-shaped elements in the blood that are essential to the process of blood clot formation, the mechanism that stops bleeding.

4. A portable battery-powered device that recognizes ventricular fibrillation and advises when a countershock is indicated. It delivers an electric shock to patients with ventricular fibrillation.

5. The _____ pulse is taken at the groin.

6. The movement of air in and out of the lungs.

9. Cessation of breathing and a heartbeat.

10. Ventricular _____ is an uncoordinated muscular quivering of the heart; the most common abnormal rhythm causing cardiac arrest.

Down

1. The wave of pressure created by the heart as it contracts and forces blood out into the major arteries.

2. Inflation of the stomach caused when excessive pressures are used during artificial ventilation and air is directed into the stomach rather than the lungs.

3. The fluid part of the blood that carries blood cells, transports nutrients, and removes cellular waste materials.

7. The _____ pulse is taken on either side of the neck.

8. The _____ pulse is located on the inside of the upper arm.

Critical Thinking

Fill-in-the-Blank

Read each item carefully and then complete the statement by filling in the missing words.

1. Chest compressions for an infant should be delivered at a rate of at least _____ per minute during CPR.

2. An infant's pulse should be checked at the _____ artery.

3. The circulatory system consists of a(n) _____, a network of pipes (the blood vessels), and _____.

4. The main artery carrying blood away from the heart is the _____.

5. _____ _____ is the temporary stiffening of muscles that occurs several hours after death.

6. Bloating of the stomach is called _____ _____.

7. Most out-of-hospital cardiac arrest patients have an irregular heart electrical rhythm called _____ _____.

8. You should practice _____ _____ when performing CPR.

9. Brain damage begins within _____ to _____ minutes after the patient has gone into cardiac arrest.

10. You should regularly update your skills by successfully completing a recognized _____ course.

Short Answer

Complete this section with short written answers using the space provided.

1. If you are using only one hand to deliver chest compressions to a child, what should you do with your other hand?

_____

_____

2. Where along the sternum should you place your fingers to deliver chest compressions to an infant?

_____

_____

3. Name two causes of gastric distention during CPR.

_____

_____

4. Name the four major arteries.

_____

_____

5. What are the four reliable signs of death?

_____

_____

6. What are the situations that you should be alerted to before operating an AED on a patient, and how do you correct them?

_____

_____

7. List the six reasons for discontinuing CPR.

_____

_____

8. What are the signs that effective CPR is being administered to the patient?

_____

_____

You Make the Call

The following scenarios provide an opportunity to explore the concerns associated with patient management. Read the scenarios and answer the questions to the best of your ability.

1. You arrive on the scene to find a 58-year-old man lying face down in his garden next to the tiller he has been operating. He does not respond to you as you approach. In fact, you think he is not breathing. What should you do?

_____

_____

_____

2. You respond to check on the well-being of an elderly woman at the request of her neighbor. The neighbor tells you that the woman is usually out in her garden every day without fail, but she has not been seen in several days. After gaining access to the woman's residence, you find her lying supine in bed. There is a foul odor in the room, and you notice that the woman is unresponsive. Your primary assessment reveals no breathing and no pulse. You observe a purplish coloring on her back. What should you do?

_____

_____

_____

Skills

Skill Drills

Skill Drill 7-1: Performing Adult Chest Compressions
Test your knowledge of this skill by filling in the correct words in the photo caption.

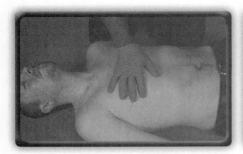
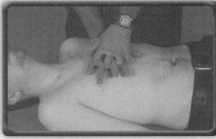
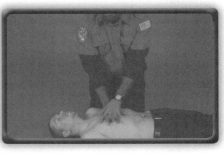

1. Locate the _____ and _____ of the sternum. Place the _____ of your hand in the center of the chest, in between the nipples.

2. Place your other hand on top of your first hand and _____ your fingers.

3. Compress the chest of an adult _____ _____ straight down.

Skill Drill 7-2: Performing One-Rescuer Adult CPR
Test your knowledge of this skill by placing the photos below in the correct order. Number the first step with a "1," the second step with a "2," etc.

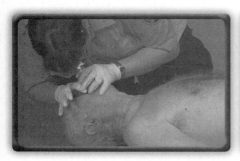
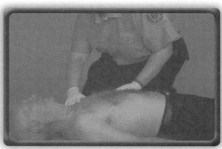
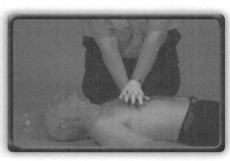

_____ Perform rescue breathing.

_____ Establish responsiveness and lack of breathing.

_____ Perform chest compressions.

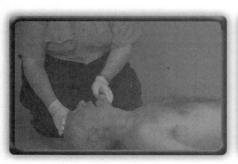
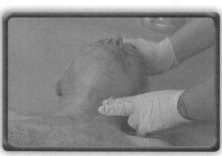

_____ Open the airway.

_____ Check for circulation.

Skill Drill 7-5: Procedure for Automated External Defibrillation
Test your knowledge of this skill by filling in the correct words in the photo caption.

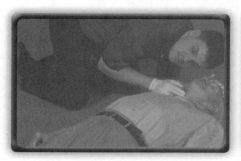

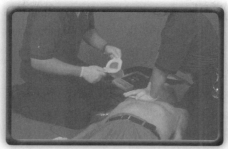

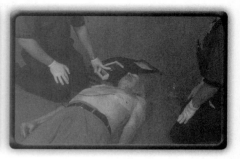

1. Check for _____,
_____, and
circulation.

2. If the patient is unresponsive, not
breathing, and _____,
begin providing chest compressions.

3. Apply the _____
_____ and connect
them to the defibrillator. Turn
on the AED. Do not touch the
_____. Allow the
AED to _____ the
rhythm.

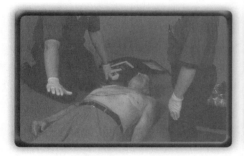

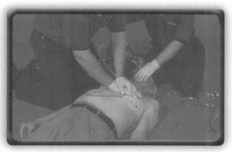

4. Determine whether a
_____ is advised
by the defibrillator. If a shock is
advised, defibrillate the patient.

5. As soon as the AED gives the shock,
perform _____
cycles of CPR (about 2 minutes),
starting with _____
_____, then analyze
the rhythm. If the AED advises
no shock, perform five cycles of
CPR (about 2 minutes), starting
with chest compressions, then
_____ the rhythm.

Patient Assessment

General Knowledge

Matching

Match each of the items in the left column to the appropriate definition in the right column.

_____ **1.** Aspiration   **A.** "What's wrong?"

_____ **2.** Auscultation   **B.** Weak pulse

_____ **3.** Bounding pulse   **C.** Listening to sounds with a stethoscope

_____ **4.** Chief complaint   **D.** Examining by touch

_____ **5.** Palpation   **E.** Head-to-toe physical examination

_____ **6.** Sign   **F.** Breathing in foreign matter

_____ **7.** Symptom   **G.** Strong pulse

_____ **8.** Thready pulse   **H.** A condition you observe in a patient

_____ **9.** Primary assessment   **I.** Assessment of airway, breathing, and circulation

_____ **10.** Secondary assessment   **J.** Something the patient tells you about his or her condition

Multiple Choice

Read each item carefully and then select the one best response.

_____ **1.** When assessing for scene safety, you should scan for:

    A. the number of injured patients.

    B. your own safety.

    C. the presence of hazards.

    D. all of the above.

_____ **2.** With patients appearing to be unconscious, you should:

    A. shout at them until they respond.

    B. shake them vigorously until they respond.

    C. call to them in a loud tone, and if you receive no response, gently touch or shake their shoulder.

    D. begin CPR immediately.

_____ **3.** If you cannot find a pulse within 5 to 10 seconds, you should:

    A. try another location.

    B. ask your partner to check.

    C. begin CPR.

    D. check the patient's skin color; if it is good, assume there is a pulse.

_____ **4.** Once an airway is open, you should do all of the following EXCEPT:

    A. immediately begin rescue breathing.

    B. clear the airway if necessary.

    C. insert an airway adjunct if necessary.

    D. check the airway for foreign bodies.

_____ **5.** When assessing respiration, you should:

    A. determine rate and quality of respiration.

    B. determine rate by checking inhalation for 30 seconds.

    C. determine quality by placing your hand over the patient's nose.

    D. tell the patient you are counting respirations and to breathe normally.

_____ **6.** Capillary refill is:

    A. tested on the patient's face.

    B. not present in children.

    C. always accurate if done correctly.

    D. the ability of the circulatory system to return blood to the capillary vessels after the blood has been squeezed out.

_____ **7.** The normal adult resting pulse rate is _____ beats per minute.

    A. 40 to 60

    B. 60 to 100

    C. 100 to 120

    D. 120 to 180

_____ **8.** The normal pulse rate for children is _____ beats per minute.

    A. 30 to 50

    B. 50 to 70

    C. 70 to 150

    D. 150 to 200

_____ **9.** During the physical examination, you should try to avoid moving which of the following parts of the body, especially in an unresponsive or injured patient?

    A. Legs

    B. Arms

    C. Neck

    D. Pelvis

_____ **10.** What is the proper order of steps in examining the extremities?

    A. Assess the circulatory status, observe the extremities, check for movement and sensation, and examine for tenderness.

    B. Assess the circulatory status, check for movement, observe the extremities, examine for tenderness, and check for sensation.

    C. Observe the extremities, examine for tenderness, check for movement and sensation, and assess the circulatory status.

    D. Observe the extremities, assess the circulatory status, check for sensation, examine for tenderness, and check for movement.

_____ **11.** The initial part of the primary assessment includes:

    A. a medical history.

    B. a SAMPLE history.

    C. a physical examination.

    D. forming a general impression.

_____ **12.** The primary assessment includes:

    A. assessing the patient's responsiveness.

    B. forming a general impression.

    C. checking ABCs.

    D. all of the above.

_____ **13.** The AVPU scale is a four-level scale used for:
   A. communicating the patient's vital signs to the hospital.
   B. describing a patient's level of consciousness.
   C. determining how rapidly you will need to transport the patient.
   D. all of the above.

_____ **14.** To check breathing:
   A. see if the chest rises and falls with each breath.
   B. place the side of your face next to the patient's nose and mouth.
   C. listen for air exchange.
   D. all of the above.

_____ **15.** To check for the brachial pulse:
   A. place your fingers halfway between the shoulder and the elbow.
   B. you need to remove the patient's shoes.
   C. you must find the patient's larynx.
   D. all of the above.

_____ **16.** The brachial pulse:
   A. is used for infants.
   B. is found on the inside of the arm.
   C. should be checked for 5 to 10 seconds.
   D. all of the above.

_____ **17.** The carotid pulse is located on the:
   A. neck.
   B. ankle.
   C. wrist.
   D. foot.

_____ **18.** The first step used to control severe bleeding is to:
   A. elevate the body part.
   B. bandage the wound.
   C. apply direct pressure.
   D. apply pressure to a pressure point.

_____ **19.** Your dispatcher should have obtained information about the:
   A. safety level of the scene.
   B. number of people involved in the incident.
   C. location of the incident.
   D. all of the above.

_____ **20.** If you can determine the mechanism of injury, you can sometimes:
   A. eliminate the need for a complete head-to-toe physical examination.
   B. predict the patient's injuries.
   C. help law enforcement officers deal with vehicle removal.
   D. all of the above.

_____ **21.** If your patient was in an automobile accident, and you notice that the windshield is broken, you should pay particular attention to the possibility of:
   A. head and spine injuries.
   B. inclement weather.
   C. chest injuries.
   D. all of the above.

_____ **22.** Yellowish skin may indicate:

    A. shock.

    B. fever or sunburn.

    C. lack of oxygen.

    D. liver problems.

_____ **23.** A blue skin tone often indicates:

    A. shock.

    B. fever or sunburn.

    C. lack of oxygen.

    D. liver problems.

_____ **24.** Flushed, reddish skin often indicates:

    A. shock.

    B. fever or sunburn.

    C. lack of oxygen.

    D. liver problems.

_____ **25.** Pale skin often indicates:

    A. shock.

    B. fever or sunburn.

    C. lack of oxygen.

    D. liver problems.

_____ **26.** When updating responding EMS units, you should include which of the following in your report?

    A. Age and sex of the patient

    B. The chief complaint

    C. Status of the airway

    D. All of the above

_____ **27.** A normal resting respiratory rate in an adult is between _____ breaths per minute.

    A. 8 and 10

    B. 12 and 20

    C. 20 and 25

    D. none of the above

_____ **28.** When you check a patient's respiratory rate:

    A. count one complete cycle of inhaling and exhaling.

    B. count for 1 minute.

    C. don't tell the patient you are counting respirations.

    D. all of the above.

_____ **29.** The capillary refill test should not be used in a cold environment because:

    A. it can delay transport.

    B. there is a higher risk of frostbite.

    C. refill will be delayed.

    D. all of the above.

_____ **30.** The patient's skin condition should be checked for all of the following EXCEPT:

    A. color.

    B. temperature.

    C. reactivity.

    D. moisture.

_____ **31.** Unequal pupils may be an indication of:

    A. stroke.

    B. cardiac arrest.

    C. diabetes.

    D. all of the above.

_____ **32.** Dilated pupils may be an indication of:

    A. cardiac arrest.

    B. the use of barbiturates.

    C. head injuries.

    D. all of the above.

_____ **33.** Pupils that remain constricted may be an indication of:

    A. cardiac arrest or head injury.

    B. stroke or brain damage.

    C. use of narcotics or central nervous system disease.

    D. none of the above.

_____ **34.** All of the following are vital signs EXCEPT:

    A. blood pressure.

    B. pulse.

    C. respiratory rate.

    D. lung sounds.

_____ **35.** A neck breather is a person who:

    A. has distended carotid veins upon exertion.

    B. has wheezing sounds when breathing.

    C. has a stoma.

    D. none of the above.

_____ **36.** Flail chest can result from:

    A. inadequate oxygen supply.

    B. multiple rib fractures.

    C. internal bleeding.

    D. all of the above.

_____ **37.** Examination of the extremities may include all of the following EXCEPT:

    A. asking the patient to move the extremity.

    B. assessing blood pressure.

    C. looking for bleeding.

    D. touching the patient's bare skin.

_____ **38.** If an adult patient is conscious, where should the pulse be assessed?

    A. Carotid artery

    B. Brachial artery

    C. Radial artery

    D. Femoral artery

_____ **39.** The purpose of obtaining a medical history is to:
  A. gather a systematic account of the patient's past medical conditions, illnesses, and injuries.
  B. gather information that can be used in court against the patient in the future.
  C. determine if the patient is psychiatrically stable.
  D. allow the patient to vent his or her concerns about the incident.

_____ **40.** When performing a secondary assessment, you should look for all of the following EXCEPT:
  A. open injuries.
  B. reflexes.
  C. deformities.
  D. swelling.

True/False

If you believe the statement to be more true than false, write the letter "T" in the space provided. If you believe the statement to be more false than true, write the letter "F."

_____ **1.** Your scene size-up begins before you arrive at the emergency scene.

_____ **2.** During the scene size-up, you should try to anticipate what equipment you need to take appropriate standard precautions.

_____ **3.** Hazards on the scene may be visible or invisible.

_____ **4.** Upon arriving at the scene, you should park your vehicle to block all traffic.

_____ **5.** The purpose of determining the mechanism of injury is to help predict patient injury.

_____ **6.** The mechanism of injury can be useful in determining all injuries that are present.

_____ **7.** AVPU is a scale used to determine level of consciousness.

_____ **8.** If patients are unconscious, it is not necessary to speak with them because they cannot hear anyway.

_____ **9.** When determining level of consciousness in infants or children, it is best to assess how they interact with their caregivers.

_____ **10.** You should always check the patient's pulse by using your thumb or index finger.

_____ **11.** The injury most readily apparent to the patient is usually the most severe injury.

_____ **12.** The head-to-toe physical examination will help you get a better picture of the patient's overall condition.

_____ **13.** You should perform the patient assessment before asking family or bystanders for information.

_____ **14.** The primary assessment is performed immediately after the scene size-up.

_____ **15.** You should take a patient's medical history before you update responding EMS units.

_____ **16.** First impressions of a patient's condition are often misleading and should therefore not be considered valuable information.

_____ **17.** One effective tool for determining a patient's responsiveness is to introduce yourself to the patient.

_____ **18.** The primary assessment is your first opportunity to check the patient's ABCs.

_____ **19.** Introducing yourself to an unconscious patient is often considered disrespectful by bystanders.

_____ **20.** If a patient is not responsive to verbal stimuli, you must assume that the airway is closed.

_____ **21.** If a patient has suffered trauma and is unconscious, use the head tilt–chin lift method to open the airway.

_____ 22. If an unconscious patient has a medical problem and has not suffered trauma, use the head tilt–chin lift method to open the airway.

_____ 23. If an adult patient is conscious, you should measure the radial pulse.

_____ 24. If an adult patient is unconscious, you should measure the carotid pulse.

_____ 25. The patient's chief complaint may be misleading but should be acknowledged anyway.

_____ 26. Downed electrical wires can be assumed to be safe if the electric company is on the scene when you arrive.

_____ 27. The head-to-toe physical examination is done to assess life-threatening conditions.

_____ 28. A sign is something about the patient you can see or feel for yourself.

_____ 29. A symptom is something the patient tells you about his or her condition.

_____ 30. The respiratory rate is the speed at which the patient is breathing.

_____ 31. The pulse indicates the speed and force with which the heart is beating.

_____ 32. The pulse can be felt anywhere on the body where an artery passes over a hard structure such as a bone.

_____ 33. The brachial pulse is used to assess the circulatory status of a leg.

_____ 34. A weak pulse is often called a threatened pulse.

_____ 35. A strong pulse is often called a bounding pulse.

_____ 36. The normal reaction of a pupil to light is to expand.

_____ 37. Swollen (distended) neck veins are usually an indication of heart problems.

_____ 38. If you suspect fractured ribs, you should avoid pushing down on the chest.

_____ 39. Rigidity is often a sign of abdominal injury.

_____ 40. If a conscious patient cannot move the foot or toes, the limb is seriously injured or paralyzed.

Labeling

Label the following diagram with the correct terms.

1. Pupil Size

A

B

C

A. _____

B. _____

C. _____

Crossword Puzzle

Use the clues in the column to complete the crossword puzzle.

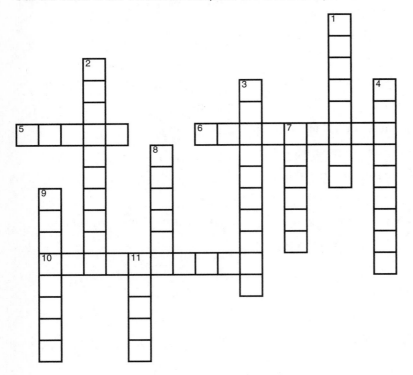

Across

5. The _____ extremity consists of the arm, forearm, wrist, and hand.

6. _____ pressure is the measurement of pressure exerted against the walls of the arteries while the left ventricle of the heart is at rest.

10. Signs of life, such as pulse, respiration, blood pressure, and skin condition.

Down

1. _____ pressure is the measurement of blood pressure exerted against the walls of the arteries during contraction of the heart.

2. _____-based care is a system of patient evaluation in which the chief complaint of the patient and other signs and symptoms are gathered. The care given is based on this information rather than on a formal diagnosis.

3. A condition that occurs when three or more ribs are each broken in two places and the chest wall lying between the fractures becomes a free-floating segment.

4. A straight board used for splinting, extricating, and transporting patients with suspected spinal injuries.

7. A wound or injury.

8. The circular openings in the middle of the eye.

9. The collarbone.

11. The _____ extremity consists of the thigh, leg, ankle, and foot.

Critical Thinking

Fill-in-the-Blank

Read each item carefully and then complete the statement by filling in the missing words.

1. The first thing you should do when determining a patient's responsiveness is to _____

_____.

2. When there is no response to verbal or painful stimuli, a patient's condition is described as _____.

3. The method for opening the airway of an unresponsive medical patient is the _____ _____–_____ _____ maneuver.

4. If a patient is responsive, assess the _____ and _____ of the patient's breathing.

5. The third part of the primary assessment is to check the _____.

6. Anything a patient tells you about his or her condition is known as a(n) _____.

7. Anything you see or feel concerning the patient's condition is known as a(n) _____.

8. A slow pulse may indicate _____ _____.

9. A fast pulse may indicate _____.

10. To assess a pulse, you should determine _____, _____, and _____.

11. Normal body temperature is _____.

12. The secondary assessment includes determining vital signs, which consist of _____, _____, _____ _____, and _____ _____.

13. Primary assessment consists of the following six steps. Arrange them in the proper order.

_____ **A.** Assess the patient's breathing.
_____ **B.** Assess the patient's responsiveness, and stabilize the spine if necessary.
_____ **C.** Form a general impression of the patient.
_____ **D.** Assess the patient's circulation, including the presence of severe bleeding.
_____ **E.** Assess the patient's airway.
_____ **F.** Update responding EMS units.

14. _____ exists when the blood pressure remains greater than 140/90 mm Hg after repeated examinations over several weeks.

15. The arrow on a blood pressure cuff should point to the _____ artery.

16. The _____ method of taking a blood pressure does not give you the diastolic pressure.

17. The first step in the reassessment of a patient is to repeat the _____ assessment.

18. The posterior tibial pulse is located just behind the ankle bone on the _____ (inner) side of the ankle.

19. Conduct a thorough, hands-on, full-body assessment in a logical, _____, systematic manner.

20. Before arriving at the scene, prepare yourself by anticipating the types of _____ _____ for infectious diseases that may be required.

Fill-in-the-Table

Fill in the missing parts of the table.

Skin Color		
Color	Term	Sign of:
Red		
White		
Blue		
Yellow		

Short Answer

Complete this section with short written answers using the space provided.

1. Name the five steps in the sequence of patient assessment.

_____

_____

2. List three pieces of information a dispatcher should obtain prior to your arrival on the scene.

_____

_____

3. List the six components of scene size-up.

_____

_____

4. List four types of hazards that may be found at any emergency scene.

_____

_____

5. List three signs to look for when determining the mechanism of injury to a patient.

_____

_____

6. What does the acronym AVPU stand for?

_____

_____

7. What is the best way to check an unresponsive patient's breathing?

_____

_____

8. What does the acronym DOTS stand for?

_____

_____

9. Describe the three pulses you will most often check, where each is located, and when each one should be used.

_____

_____

10. Describe the method for checking capillary refill.

_____

_____

11. What does the acronym SAMPLE stand for?

_____

_____

12. Describe the proper sequence of body areas to check in the full-body assessment of a patient.

_____

_____

13. List four places to look for skin color changes in patients with deeply pigmented skin.

_____

_____

14. List the eight components of the hand-off report to an EMS unit.

_____

_____

_____

You Make the Call

The following scenarios provide an opportunity to explore the concerns associated with patient management. Read the scenarios and answer the questions to the best of your ability.

1. You are dispatched to a residence for an 83-year-old woman who is reportedly unconscious. As you arrive, the woman's husband tells you he thinks she has had a stroke. What should you do?

_____

_____

_____

2. You are on the scene of a 55-year-old man experiencing chest pain. The EMT on scene would like to assist the patient with some nitroglycerin and needs a blood pressure reading before he administers the medication. The EMT hands you the blood pressure cuff and asks you to obtain a reading. What should you do?

_____

_____

_____

Medical Emergencies

General Knowledge

Matching

Match each of the items in the left column to the appropriate definition in the right column.

_____ **1.** Diabetic coma

_____ **2.** Bronchitis

_____ **3.** Asthma

_____ **4.** Stroke

_____ **5.** Acute abdomen

_____ **6.** Dyspnea

_____ **7.** Insulin shock

_____ **8.** Absence seizures

_____ **9.** Chronic obstructive pulmonary disease (COPD)

_____ **10.** Angina pectoris

A. Caused by an inadequate flow of blood to heart muscle

B. Inflammation of the airways in the lungs

C. Caused by chronic bronchial obstruction (emphysema)

D. Difficulty or pain with breathing

E. Sudden onset of abdominal pain caused by disease or trauma

F. Blood clot or a broken blood vessel in the brain

G. Disease that causes narrowing and inflammation of the airways

H. Occurs when the body has too much blood glucose and not enough insulin

I. Occurs if the body has enough insulin but not enough blood glucose

J. Brief lapse of attention

Multiple Choice

Read each item carefully and then select the one best response.

_____ **1.** An acute abdomen is:

   A. irritated or infected.

   B. healthy.

   C. caused by overeating.

   D. large.

_____ **2.** Which of the following heart conditions rarely lasts more than 5 minutes and is usually relieved when the patient takes a nitroglycerin pill?

   A. Heart attack

   B. Cardiac arrest

   C. Angina pectoris

   D. Congestive heart failure

_____ **3.** If the heart becomes weak and does not pump properly, the patient will most likely experience:

   A. cardiac arrest.

   B. crushing chest pain.

   C. congestion of blood in the heart, which causes the heart to stop pumping.

   D. congestion of the blood vessels of the lungs, which causes breathing difficulties.

_____ **4.** Complete blockage of an artery in the heart by a blood clot or a buildup of fatty deposits will result in:
- **A.** chest pain.
- **B.** heart attack.
- **C.** atherosclerosis.
- **D.** breathing difficulties.

_____ **5.** The first step in caring for a patient who has chest pain should be to:
- **A.** begin CPR.
- **B.** assist the patient in contacting a physician.
- **C.** examine the patient for chest wounds.
- **D.** summon additional help.

_____ **6.** A man who tells you that he feels as if something is sitting on, pressing on, or crushing his chest is most likely having a heart attack or:
- **A.** a stroke.
- **B.** cardiac arrest.
- **C.** an angina attack.
- **D.** congestive heart failure.

_____ **7.** If you suspect or cannot tell whether a person is having a heart attack, your first concern should be to:
- **A.** call for additional help.
- **B.** make the person comfortable.
- **C.** place the person on a hard surface.
- **D.** try to relieve the person's pain by giving them aspirin.

_____ **8.** Your second concern for a patient believed to be having a heart attack should be to:
- **A.** call for additional help.
- **B.** make the person comfortable.
- **C.** place the person on a hard surface.
- **D.** try to relieve the person's emotional distress.

_____ **9.** If a patient having a heart attack goes into cardiac arrest, you should first:
- **A.** begin CPR.
- **B.** give oxygen.
- **C.** try to make the patient comfortable.
- **D.** transport the patient to the hospital.

_____ **10.** The first step in caring for patients who are having difficulty breathing is to:
- **A.** check for airway obstruction.
- **B.** put them in a comfortable position to ease breathing.
- **C.** ask them if they are being treated for a heart condition.
- **D.** ask if they are experiencing chest pain.

_____ **11.** Which of the following statements regarding asthma is false?
- **A.** Asthma involves acute spasm of the smaller air passages.
- **B.** Patients can have great difficulty exhaling.
- **C.** Pursed-lip breathing offers no benefit.
- **D.** Wheezing lung sounds can be heard.

_____ **12.** The first priority in treating a stroke patient is to:
- **A.** give the patient emotional support.
- **B.** determine if the patient is paralyzed.
- **C.** maintain the airway and give oxygen, if possible.
- **D.** arrange for prompt transportation to the hospital.

_____ **13.** The second priority in treating a stroke patient is to:

    A. maintain the airway.

    B. watch for convulsions.

    C. provide emotional support.

    D. arrange for prompt transportation to the hospital.

_____ **14.** The Cincinnati Prehospital Stroke Scale measures which of the following?

    A. Facial droop, arm drift, abnormal speech

    B. Facial balance, arm strength, hearing

    C. All of the above

    D. None of the above

_____ **15.** Insulin is best described as:

    A. a substance similar to glucose.

    B. a chemical that is injected to counteract insulin shock.

    C. a chemical that allows glucose in the blood to be used as fuel in the body's cells.

    D. a diabetic medication for patients who cannot produce glucose in their blood.

_____ **16.** A person with diabetes has abnormally low levels of insulin in the body and, as a result, must:

    A. always wear a medical alert tag.

    B. eat more sugar than most.

    C. avoid eating sugar in any form.

    D. supplement insulin levels with insulin injections or oral medication.

_____ **17.** A person in insulin shock must receive:

    A. CPR.

    B. glucose.

    C. insulin.

    D. oxygen.

_____ **18.** The signs and symptoms of insulin shock should be considered:

    A. similar to those of other types of shock.

    B. more serious than those of a diabetic coma.

    C. different from those of other types of shock.

    D. almost impossible to identify unless the person is wearing a medical alert tag.

_____ **19.** Which of the following systems are located in the abdomen?

    A. Circulatory

    B. Digestive

    C. Genitourinary

    D. All of the above

_____ **20.** All of the following regarding an acute abdomen are true EXCEPT:

    A. the abdomen may be hard as a board.

    B. the patient may experience diarrhea.

    C. it may be caused by an aneurysm.

    D. the patient may complain of frequent urination.

_____ **21.** Which of the following is not considered a risk factor for an abdominal aortic aneurysm?

    A. Smoking

    B. Hypertension

    C. Angina

    D. Diabetes

_____ **22.** Your first step in caring for a patient with an abdominal aortic aneurysm should be to:
  A. place the patient on his or her back.
  B. place the patient in a comfortable position and arrange for prompt transport.
  C. administer nitroglycerin.
  D. give the patient something to eat and drink.

_____ **23.** A patient with chronic renal failure:
  A. is still able to filter waste from his or her bloodstream.
  B. experiences increases in blood pressure after hemodialysis.
  C. typically must receive dialysis daily.
  D. may have a shunt implanted in his or her arm for hemodialysis.

_____ **24.** The patient assessment sequence does not include the use of:
  A. ABCs.
  B. a physical examination.
  C. CPR.
  D. SAMPLE.

_____ **25.** If a patient is seizing on a hard surface, the EMR can:
  A. restrain the patient.
  B. keep the patient's airway open.
  C. assess the level of consciousness.
  D. place his or her feet under the patient's head.

_____ **26.** The letters in SAMPLE will help an EMR to remember the steps of:
  A. conducting a physical examination.
  B. collecting a medical history.
  C. assessing an accident scene.
  D. performing CPR.

_____ **27.** Once a seizure has stopped, the first action of the EMR is to:
  A. begin CPR.
  B. ensure an open airway.
  C. assess the patient's level of consciousness.
  D. gather the patient's medical history.

_____ **28.** An important reason for an EMR to locate a patient's dialysis shunt is:
  A. to assess it for blood clots.
  B. to make sure a blood pressure reading is obtained in the opposite arm.
  C. to determine how often the patient receives dialysis.
  D. none of the above.

_____ **29.** A patient complaining of tearing abdominal pain accompanied with shoulder pain may be experiencing a(n):
  A. abdominal aortic aneurysm.
  B. heart attack.
  C. stroke.
  D. none of the above.

_____ **30.** A patient experiencing a diabetic coma:
  A. may appear intoxicated.
  B. may appear to have the flu.
  C. produces too much insulin.
  D. should not be given oral glucose.

_____ **31.** Which of the following statements regarding strokes is false?

    A. Signs and symptoms can vary depending on what part of the brain is affected.

    B. Some stroke patients experience seizures.

    C. People with low blood pressure have an increased risk of stroke.

    D. Some stroke patients are unable to speak.

_____ **32.** All of the following are signs of a stroke EXCEPT:

    A. tightness in the chest.

    B. numbness on one side of the body.

    C. dizziness.

    D. respiratory arrest.

_____ **33.** Layers of fat can coat the inner walls of the arteries, causing them to become narrower. This process:

    A. is called atherosclerosis.

    B. causes angina pectoris.

    C. causes heart attacks.

    D. all of the above.

_____ **34.** Which of the following statements regarding angina pectoris is false?

    A. It may cause fear and a sense of doom.

    B. It may be treated with nitroglycerin.

    C. It may cause pain in the arms, neck, or jaw.

    D. It may cause severe abdominal pain.

_____ **35.** Nitroglycerin should:

    A. not be taken at intervals of less than 10 minutes.

    B. be given by mouth or in aerosol form.

    C. always ease the pain of a heart attack.

    D. all of the above.

_____ **36.** A heart attack:

    A. is known as a myocardial infarction.

    B. is caused by complete blockage of a coronary artery.

    C. causes part of the heart muscle to die.

    D. all of the above.

_____ **37.** A patient is short of breath, weak, sweating, nauseated, and complains of crushing pain from the chest to the left arm or jaw. The EMR should:

    A. call for additional help.

    B. talk to the patient to reassure him or her and establish a bond with the patient.

    C. help the patient find a comfortable position.

    D. all of the above.

_____ **38.** The heart is not pumping adequately, and the circulatory system becomes unbalanced. Which of the following statements applies?

    A. The patient will be short of breath.

    B. The patient will complain of crushing chest pain.

    C. CPR should be provided.

    D. All of the above.

_____ **39.** Shortness of breath, rapid and shallow breathing, moist or gurgling respirations, profuse sweating, and swollen ankles are all signs and symptoms of:

    A. cardiac arrest.

    B. myocardial infarction.

    C. congestive heart failure.

    D. diabetic coma.

_____ **40.** Treatment of a patient with congestive heart failure includes:

    A. placing the legs lower than the rest of the body.

    B. administering nitroglycerin.

    C. CPR.

    D. all of the above.

_____ **41.** A diabetic who has taken insulin but has not eaten enough food may:

    A. experience insulin shock.

    B. become dizzy or confused.

    C. have pale, moist, cool skin and a rapid pulse.

    D. all of the above.

_____ **42.** A state of sickness that occurs when the body has too much glucose and not enough insulin is:

    A. diabetes.

    B. insulin shock.

    C. diabetic coma.

    D. none of the above.

_____ **43.** A disease in which the body is unable to use glucose normally because of a deficiency or total lack of insulin is:

    A. diabetes.

    B. insulin shock.

    C. diabetic coma.

    D. none of the above.

_____ **44.** Insulin shock can:

    A. be treated with glucose.

    B. occur quickly.

    C. be confused with drunkenness.

    D. all of the above.

_____ **45.** A rapid, weak pulse; deep, rapid breathing; and a history of diabetes are signs and symptoms of:

    A. a diabetic coma.

    B. too much blood glucose in the body.

    C. failure to take insulin over a period of days.

    D. all of the above.

True/False

If you believe the statement to be more true than false, write the letter "T" in the space provided. If you believe the statement to be more false than true, write the letter "F."

_____ **1.** The emergency medical care that EMRs can provide to people who have heart attacks sometimes saves their lives.

_____ **2.** One seizure typically lasts between 30 and 45 minutes.

_____ **3.** If a person is having a seizure, you should attempt to apply restraints.

_____ **4.** A person who is anxious or hostile after a seizure may be embarrassed and need privacy.

_____ **5.** A person having a seizure should only be moved if he or she is in a dangerous location.

_____ **6.** If a person is having a seizure, you should place a barrier between his or her teeth.

_____ **7.** Some seizures may have serious underlying causes such as stroke or diabetic emergencies.

_____ **8.** Patients are usually responsive during seizures.

_____ **9.** You cannot adequately ventilate a nonbreathing patient during a seizure.

_____ **10.** A person in a diabetic coma needs insulin.

_____ **11.** Even if you are unsure about whether a fully responsive patient is in a diabetic coma or insulin shock, you can give glucose without harming the patient.

_____ **12.** A person who has had a stroke may appear unresponsive yet still be able to hear you.

_____ **13.** The only way for responders to care for stroke patients is by providing oxygen.

_____ **14.** A blood clot or a rupture of a blood vessel anywhere in the body can cause a stroke.

_____ **15.** Symptoms of a stroke can vary because different areas of the brain can be affected by a stroke.

_____ **16.** Stroke patients are always unresponsive.

_____ **17.** Unequal pupil size and difficulty speaking are two common signs of stroke.

_____ **18.** A person who has had a severe stroke may stop breathing.

_____ **19.** A patient with abdominal pain should be examined by a physician.

_____ **20.** It is necessary to determine the exact cause of a medical problem before appropriate treatment can be administered.

_____ **21.** During a seizure, if the patient stops breathing and turns blue, CPR should be administered.

_____ **22.** Many factors cause seizures, and the type of seizure will indicate the cause.

_____ **23.** The AVPU scale is used to assess a patient's mental status and may be used when there has been a head injury, poisoning, or an infection.

_____ **24.** An EMR must first determine the cause of the patient's altered level of consciousness and then begin appropriate treatment.

_____ **25.** It is important to categorize patients as only medical patients or trauma patients to determine the best course of treatment.

_____ **26.** Chest pain with squeezing or tightness in the chest may be a sign of angina pectoris.

_____ **27.** Exertion, emotion, or eating can contribute to angina attacks.

_____ **28.** Causes of dyspnea include angina pectoris, heart attack, congestive heart failure, chronic obstructive lung disease, emphysema, chronic bronchitis, and pneumonia.

_____ **29.** It is important to determine the cause of dyspnea so as to determine the appropriate treatment.

_____ **30.** Loosening any tight clothing and comfortably positioning the patient are steps in treatment for a patient with dyspnea.

Crossword Puzzle

Use the clues in the column to complete the crossword puzzle.

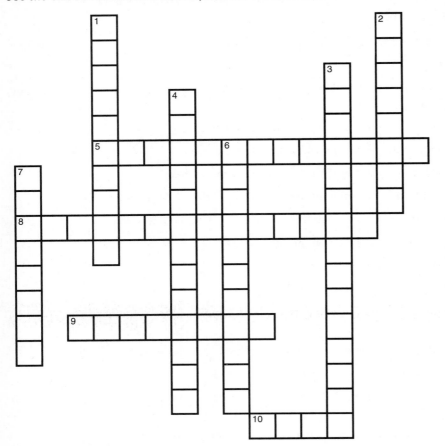

Across

5. A medication used to treat angina pectoris; increases blood flow and oxygen supply to the heart muscle and reduces or eliminates the pain of angina pectoris.

8. An abdominal _____ is a condition in which the layers of the aorta in the abdomen weaken. This causes blood to leak between the layers of the artery, causing it to bulge and sometimes rupture.

9. Do not attempt to _____ a patient during a seizure, as you may cause further injury.

10. Progression from insulin shock to a diabetic coma usually takes several _____.

Down

1. The _____ Prehospital Stroke Scale is used to determine whether a patient may have experienced a stroke.

2. Patients experiencing CHF may make a(n) _____ sound when breathing and start spitting up a white or pink froth or foamy fluid.

3. A disease characterized by a thickening and destruction of the arterial walls and caused by fatty deposits within them; the arteries lose the ability to dilate and carry blood.

4. Sudden cessation of heart function.

6. _____ seizures produce shaking movements and involve the entire body; also called grand mal seizures.

7. A disease in which the body is unable to use glucose normally because of a deficiency or total lack of insulin.

Critical Thinking

Fill-in-the-Blank

Read each item carefully and then complete the statement by filling in the missing words.

1. Altered _____ status is a sudden or gradual decrease in the patient's level of responsiveness.

2. Coronary arteries may narrow as a result of a disease process called _____, in which layers of fat coat the inner walls of the arteries.

3. _____ are caused by sudden episodes of uncontrolled electrical impulses in the brain.

4. Patients experiencing a(n) _____ _____ have great difficulty exhaling through partially obstructed air passages.

5. Following a seizure, the patient will experience a state of confusion that may last for _____ to _____ minutes.

6. When you are assessing altered mental status, remember to use the _____ scale.

7. COPD and _____ are caused by damage to the small air sacs (alveoli) in the lungs.

8. _____ are the leading cause of brain injury and disability in adults.

9. A(n) _____ is a surgically created connection between an artery and a vein.

10. A(n) _____ _____ is caused by irritation of the abdominal wall.

Fill-in-the-Table

Fill in the missing parts of the table.

Comparing Insulin Shock and Diabetic Coma	
Insulin Shock	**Diabetic Coma**
_____, _____, _____ skin	_____, _____ skin
_____, _____ pulse	_____ pulse
_____ breathing	_____, _____ breathing
Dizziness or headache	—
_____ or unconsciousness	_____ or unconsciousness
_____ onset of symptoms (_____)	_____ onset of symptoms (_____)

Short Answer

Complete this section with short written answers using the space provided.

1. Describe two medical emergencies that can occur as a result of diabetes.

_____

_____

2. What three questions should you ask a person who you believe is going into insulin shock?

_____

_____

3. Name three substances with high concentrations of glucose that would be appropriate to give to a person in insulin shock.

_____

_____

4. When assessing the patient's mental status, what two factors should be considered?

_____

_____

5. List four conditions that may contribute to an altered level of consciousness.

_____

_____

6. List five signs and symptoms of congestive heart failure.

_____

_____

7. What are the three areas of assessment when using the Cincinnati Prehospital Stroke Scale?

_____

_____

You Make the Call

The following scenarios provide an opportunity to explore the concerns associated with patient management. Read the scenarios and answer the questions to the best of your ability.

1. When you arrive at the grocery store, you are greeted by a young woman asking you to help her mother. As you are walking to the mother, the young woman explains that her mother, who is a diabetic, became confused and is now unresponsive. When you complete your AVPU assessment, you find she responds only to pain. What should you do?

_____

_____

_____

2. You respond to a call for trouble breathing. When you arrive, you find a 75-year-old man struggling to breathe. You notice he has gurgling sounds when breathing, and he is coughing up pink fluid. The patient has swollen ankles, and he tells you he had a heart attack 6 months ago. What should you do?

_____

_____

_____

Poisoning and Substance Abuse

General Knowledge

Matching

Match each of the items in the left column to the appropriate definition in the right column.

_____ **1.** Carbon monoxide

_____ **2.** Cocaine

_____ **3.** Amphetamines

_____ **4.** Hallucinogens

_____ **5.** Central nervous system

_____ **6.** Toxic

_____ **7.** Barbiturates

_____ **8.** Hives

_____ **9.** Acid

_____ **10.** Coma

A. Identified as poisonous

B. State of consciousness from which the patient cannot be aroused

C. Includes the brain and spinal cord

D. Chemical substance with a pH of less than 7.0 that can cause severe burns

E. Depressants of the nervous system

F. Powerful stimulant that induces an extreme state of euphoria

G. Colorless, odorless, poisonous gas formed by incomplete combustion

H. Allergic skin disorder marked by patches of swelling, redness, and intense itching

I. Drugs that stimulate the central nervous system

J. Chemicals that cause a person to see visions or hear sounds that are not real

Multiple Choice

Read each item carefully and then select the one best response.

_____ **1.** More than _____ of all poisonings are caused by ingestion.

    A. 50%

    B. 80%

    C. 90%

    D. 65%

_____ **2.** Which of the following statements regarding ammonia is false?

    A. It is used as fertilizer.

    B. SCBA is not required when entering an area that contains ammonia.

    C. It can severely burn the skin.

    D. It has an irritating odor.

_____ **3.** Activated charcoal:

    A. is a finely ground powder mixed with milk to make it easier to swallow.

    B. is typically given in doses of 12.5 to 25 g for adults.

    C. binds to poisons, preventing absorption in the digestive tract.

    D. is used when patients have ingested an acid or base.

_____ **4.** The first step in treating a patient who has inhaled any poison gas is to:

    A. identify the gas that is present.

    B. remove the patient from the source of the gas.

    C. transport the patient to the closest facility.

    D. call the poison control center for direction.

_____ **5.** Your patient has been poisoned by absorption. You should first:

    A. administer supplementary oxygen.

    B. wash the affected area.

    C. treat for shock.

    D. have the patient remove his or her clothing, then brush off the dry chemical.

_____ **6.** After removing chemicals absorbed into clothing, responders treating patients poisoned by absorption should:

    A. arrange for immediate transport to the hospital.

    B. wash the patient thoroughly with a hose or a shower.

    C. ask the patient to lie down and then elevate his or her legs.

    D. withhold any additional treatment unless the person feels dizzy.

_____ **7.** When caring for a patient experiencing hallucinations, you should do all of the following EXCEPT:

    A. try to reduce auditory and visual stimulation.

    B. provide the patient with auditory and visual stimulation.

    C. avoid the use of bright lights and loud noises.

    D. approach the emergency scene with caution.

_____ **8.** What medicine is used to treat anaphylactic shock?

    A. Pralidoxime chloride

    B. Benadryl

    C. Epinephrine

    D. Atropine

_____ **9.** If poison enters the body through the mouth and is absorbed by the digestive system, it is called:

    A. inhalation.

    B. ingestion.

    C. injection.

    D. absorption.

_____ **10.** If a poison enters the body through the mouth or nose and is absorbed by the mucous membranes lining the respiratory system, it is called:

    A. inhalation.

    B. ingestion.

    C. injection.

    D. absorption.

_____ **11.** When poison enters the body through a small opening in the skin, it may then be spread by the circulatory system. This is known as:

    A. inhalation.

    B. ingestion.

    C. absorption.

    D. injection.

_____ **12.** If poison enters the body through intact skin, it may then be spread by the circulatory system. This is known as:

    A. inhalation.

    B. ingestion.

    C. absorption.

    D. injection.

_____ **13.** Signs and symptoms of poisoning by ingestion may include all of the following EXCEPT:

    A. abdominal pain and diarrhea.

    B. nausea and vomiting.

    C. unusual breath odors.

    D. chest tightness.

_____ **14.** The first step in treating a patient who has ingested a poison is to:

    A. induce vomiting.

    B. dilute the poison with water.

    C. administer activated charcoal.

    D. attempt to identify the poison.

_____ **15.** Syrup of ipecac:

    A. will induce vomiting.

    B. requires a prescription.

    C. can be administered safely for any type of poisoning.

    D. is typically used in unresponsive patients.

_____ **16.** Which of the following is not one of the four kinds of poisonous snakes found in the United States?

    A. Cottonmouth

    B. Garter snake

    C. Copperhead

    D. Rattlesnake

_____ **17.** Respiratory distress, cough, dizziness, headache, and confusion may be signs of poisoning by:

    A. ingestion.

    B. inhalation.

    C. injection.

    D. absorption.

_____ **18.** If several members of one household are found at home, all with headache, nausea, disorientation, or unconsciousness, you should:

    A. remove everyone from the dwelling.

    B. suspect carbon monoxide poisoning.

    C. administer oxygen if available.

    D. all of the above.

_____ **19.** Your first priority when arriving at the scene of a call involving a suspected nerve agent should be:

    A. supporting the airway, breathing, and circulation of patients.

    B. administering antidote to patients exhibiting nerve agent symptoms.

    C. evacuating patients for at least 10 minutes until the gases dissipate.

    D. keeping yourself and others around you from becoming contaminated.

_____ **20.** Which of the following is not a sign of anaphylactic shock?

    A. Itching, hives, and swelling

    B. Rapid, shallow breathing

    C. Increased blood pressure

    D. Wheezing

_____ **21.** Which of the following statements regarding abuse of inhalants is true?

    A. It should be treated with low-flow oxygen.

    B. It can cause slowing of the heart rate.

    C. It can lead to unconsciousness and death.

    D. It is more common among adults.

_____ **22.** Which of the following statements regarding patients who have absorbed poisons is false?

    A. They may have been in contact with insecticides or industrial chemicals.

    B. They may have skin irritation.

    C. They may exhibit signs and symptoms such as nausea, vomiting, dizziness, or shock.

    D. The affected area should be immediately washed with water.

_____ **23.** Delirium tremens (DTs):

   A. are a common side effect of snake-bite treatment.

   B. usually only occur in children and adolescents.

   C. are a serious and possibly fatal medical emergency.

   D. usually appear 7 to 10 days after a person stops drinking.

_____ **24.** Drugs that stimulate the nervous system:

   A. include PCP and LSD.

   B. include amphetamines and cocaine.

   C. include opiates and marijuana.

   D. all of the above.

_____ **25.** An EMR's responsibility in a call involving drug overdose includes:

   A. providing basic life support.

   B. keeping the patient from hurting himself or herself and others.

   C. arranging for prompt transport to a medical facility.

   D. all of the above.

True/False

If you believe the statement to be more true than false, write the letter "T" in the space provided. If you believe the statement to be more false than true, write the letter "F."

_____ **1.** Accidental poisoning is most common among teenagers.

_____ **2.** Many overdoses are the result of mixing alcohol with other drugs.

_____ **3.** Most ingested poisons can be diluted by giving the patient water to drink, provided he or she is conscious and able to swallow.

_____ **4.** With ingested poisons, treat the patient, then immediately attempt to identify the substance taken.

_____ **5.** Ipecac is a nonharmful drug and can be used as a treatment for all ingested poisons.

_____ **6.** The history of the patient and of the incident as well as visual clues are important in determining appropriate treatment of a patient who may have been poisoned.

_____ **7.** More than half of all poisoning cases are caused by injection.

_____ **8.** Signs of delirium tremens include shaking, restlessness, and confusion.

_____ **9.** Treatment of anaphylactic shock involves the use of a DuoDote kit.

_____ **10.** Activated charcoal should be placed under the tongue of an unconscious patient who may have been poisoned.

_____ **11.** The EMR life support kit should contain the number of the poison control center.

_____ **12.** A tongue depressor should be used to induce vomiting in an unconscious patient who has been poisoned.

_____ **13.** If a patient shows signs and symptoms of poisoning but the poison cannot be identified easily, the safest treatment is to induce vomiting.

_____ **14.** A substance that causes poisoning by inhalation will always irritate the lungs and cause respiratory distress.

_____ **15.** A large quantity of carbon monoxide must be present for poisoning to occur.

_____ **16.** In agricultural settings, poisoning by chlorine gas is likely to occur and requires the use of a proper encapsulating suit with an SCBA.

_____ **17.** Activated charcoal is safe to use with any ingestion of poison.

_____ **18.** Animal stings and bites are one type of poisoning by injection.

_____ **19.** Poisoning by injection only includes the use of illegal drugs.

_____ **20.** Injected poisons may cause an anaphylactic reaction.

_____ **21.** Snake bite is the second leading cause of fatalities in rural areas of the United States.

_____ **22.** Permanent injury may result from snake bites.

_____ **23.** Shock, nausea, vomiting, sweating, and fainting may all be signs and symptoms of snake bite.

_____ **24.** Shock, dizziness, itching, burning, skin rash, and inflammation or redness of the skin may all be signs and symptoms of poisoning by absorption.

_____ **25.** Treatment of a patient who has absorbed a poisonous substance should begin by ensuring that the patient is no longer in contact with the toxic substance.

_____ **26.** Treatment of a patient who has absorbed a poisonous substance may require removal of the patient's clothes, followed immediately by a complete washing of the patient's body with large amounts of water.

_____ **27.** In cases of absorbed chemicals, the patient should be treated for any symptoms, shock, and breathing difficulties, if observed.

_____ **28.** Uppers such as amphetamines and cocaine are the most commonly abused drugs in our society.

_____ **29.** Auto accidents cause twice as many deaths as alcohol abuse.

_____ **30.** A well-trained and knowledgeable EMR will easily differentiate the symptoms of alcohol intoxication from those of insulin shock, diabetic coma, and other drug reactions.

_____ **31.** Users of hallucinogens may feel no pain, so they may be in danger of injuring themselves.

Crossword Puzzle

Use the clues in the column to complete the crossword puzzle.

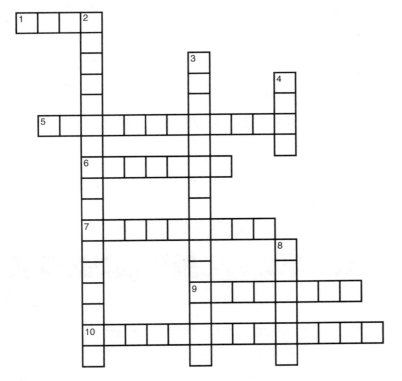

Across

1. A complete unit for delivery of air to a rescuer who enters a contaminated area; contains a mask, regulator, and air supply.

5. These should be brushed off a patient before any contact with water is made.

6. Has a strong and irritating odor, can burn the skin, and requires use of a proper encapsulating suit with an SCBA.

7. The most common method of poisoning.

9. Used to treat poisoning from a nerve agent.

10. Combines with red blood cells more readily than oxygen.

Down

2. Severe shock caused by an allergic reaction to food, medicine, or insect stings.

3. A severe, often fatal, complication of alcohol withdrawal that most commonly occurs 3 to 4 days after withdrawal (though it can occur as late as 10 days after withdrawal). It is characterized by restlessness, fever, sweating, confusion, disorientation, agitation, hallucinations, and convulsions.

4. A chemical with a pH of greater than 7.0; also called caustics or alkalis.

8. Any substance that may cause injury or death if relatively small amounts are ingested, inhaled, absorbed, applied to, or injected into the body.

Critical Thinking

Fill-in-the-Blank

Read each item carefully and then complete the statement by filling in the missing words.

1. Poisons may be ingested, inhaled, absorbed, or injected. For each of the following findings, indicate which type of poisoning has occurred.

    _____   **A.** Stains around the mouth
    _____   **B.** A group of unconscious people in a house in the winter
    _____   **C.** The smell of bleach
    _____   **D.** Swelling with red streaks radiating from it
    _____   **E.** Empty pill bottles
    _____   **F.** A worker at a water treatment plant having difficulty breathing
    _____   **G.** A worker at a dry chemical plant who is dizzy

2. Many gases irritate the respiratory tract. Two of the most frequently encountered irritating gases are _____ and _____.

3. Identify whether each of the following is associated with amphetamines (A), barbiturates (B), or hallucinogens (H).

    _____   **A.** PCP or mescaline
    _____   **B.** Overdose symptoms include talkativeness and restlessness
    _____   **C.** Tranquilizers
    _____   **D.** Overdose symptoms include respiratory depression or respiratory arrest.
    _____   **E.** LSD or peyote
    _____   **F.** Cocaine or crack
    _____   **G.** Overdose symptoms include seeing or hearing things that are not real

4. The most popularly abused drugs fall into four categories: amphetamines, barbiturates, hallucinogens, and _____.

5. A patient who has attempted _____ needs both medical and psychological support.

Fill-in-the-Table

Fill in the missing parts of the table.

Symptoms of Exposure to an Organophosphate Insecticide or Nerve Agent	
S	
L	
U	
D	
G	
E	

Short Answer

Complete this section with short written answers using the space provided.

1. Identify the most common method of poisoning.

_____

_____

2. Identify the result of administering syrup of ipecac to a patient who shows signs and symptoms of poisoning.

_____

_____

3. Name five common signs of inhalation poisoning.

_____

_____

4. What should you do if several members of one household are found at home, all experiencing headache, nausea, disorientation, or unconsciousness?

_____

_____

5. What safety equipment does ammonia contamination require?

_____

_____

6. Name three commons signs or symptoms of anaphylactic shock.

_____

_____

7. Name four commons signs or symptoms of poisoning by absorption.

_____

_____

8. What are an EMR's responsibilities in a situation of drug overdose?

_____

_____

9. In situations of poisoning by absorption, dry chemicals should be brushed off a patient before what step of care is taken?

_____

_____

You Make the Call

The following scenarios provide an opportunity to explore the concerns associated with patient management. Read the scenarios and answer the questions to the best of your ability.

1. Your neighbor comes running to your home for help. She is sure her 3-year-old has taken several pills from the bathroom medicine cabinet, thinking they were candy. The child is becoming very sleepy by the time you arrive. What should you do?

   _____

   _____

   _____

2. You are called in the middle of the night to a residence for an unknown alarm. Upon arrival, you see a family of four standing on the front lawn and hear a smoke detector alarm coming from the house. The mother tells you the alarm woke them, and they immediately exited the home. The father and two children are complaining of headaches. They are unsure why the alarm is sounding. You see no signs of smoke coming from the residence. What should you do?

   _____

   _____

   _____

Behavioral Emergencies

General Knowledge

Matching

Match each of the items in the left column to the appropriate definition in the right column.

_____ 1. Redirection	A. Mental disturbance characterized by defective or lack of contact with reality
_____ 2. Situational crisis	B. Means of focusing the patient's attention on the immediate situation or crisis
_____ 3. Emotional shock	C. Rephrasing a patient's own statement to show that he or she is being heard and understood by the rescuer
_____ 4. Critical incident stress debriefing (CISD)	D. State of emotional upset or turmoil caused by a sudden and disruptive event
_____ 5. Behavioral emergency	E. Self-inflicted death
_____ 6. Posttraumatic stress disorder (PTSD)	F. State of shock caused by sudden illness, accident, or the death of a loved one
_____ 7. Empathy	G. Ability to participate in another person's feelings or ideas
_____ 8. Suicide	H. System of psychological support designed to reduce stress on emergency personnel
_____ 9. Restatement	I. Patient exhibits abnormal behavior that is unacceptable and cannot be tolerated
_____ 10. Psychotic behavior	J. Symptoms include flashbacks to a traumatic event, depression, sleep disturbances, and guilt

Multiple Choice

Read each item carefully and then select the one best response.

_____ 1. Which of the following is not one of the phases of situational crisis?
- **A.** Anger
- **B.** Grief
- **C.** Acceptance
- **D.** Emotional shock

_____ 2. You arrive at the scene of a motor vehicle crash and find a teenage girl staring at other emergency personnel caring for an older woman. She then says, "If I hadn't asked her to take me to the mall, this wouldn't have happened." What phase of a situational crisis is this girl probably experiencing?
- **A.** Anxiety
- **B.** Denial
- **C.** Remorse
- **D.** Emotional shock

_____ 3. Which of the following should you not do when talking to a patient?
- **A.** Establish eye contact.
- **B.** Bring yourself to the patient's level.
- **C.** Talk in a calm, steady voice.
- **D.** Tell the patient that everything will be all right, if it will make the patient feel better.

_____   **4.** _____ responder(s) should attempt to talk to a potentially violent person.

    A. One

    B. Two

    C. No

    D. Any number of

_____   **5.** What is the correct order of the phases of the domestic abuse cycle?

    A. Explosive, make up, tension

    B. Tension, make up, explosive

    C. Make up, tension, explosive

    D. Tension, explosive, make up

_____   **6.** All of the following are true regarding behavioral emergencies EXCEPT:

    A. They may be caused by situational stress or physical trauma.

    B. They are not caused by injuries such as head trauma.

    C. They call for appropriate communication, especially body language.

    D. They describe situations where people behave in an abnormal and unacceptable manner.

_____   **7.** Behavioral emergencies are caused by:

    A. over-the-counter medications.

    B. situational stresses.

    C. uncontrolled diabetes or respiratory conditions.

    D. all of the above.

_____   **8.** A person experiencing a situational crisis may go through which emotional phases?

    A. Denial or anger

    B. Psychotic phase

    C. Anaphylactic shock

    D. All of the above

_____   **9.** A person who is experiencing high anxiety is likely to exhibit all of the following characteristics EXCEPT:

    A. a loud or screaming voice.

    B. frustration and anger.

    C. rapid breathing and rapid speech.

    D. a calm demeanor.

_____   **10.** Emotional shock may:

    A. cause the patient to have warm, dry skin.

    B. cause a strong, fast pulse.

    C. cause vomiting and nausea.

    D. all of the above.

_____   **11.** Rephrasing a patient's own statement to show understanding is called:

    A. empathy.

    B. redirection.

    C. restatement.

    D. counter-phrasing.

_____   **12.** A means of focusing the patient's attention on the immediate situation or crisis is called:

    A. empathy.

    B. redirection.

    C. restatement.

    D. counter-phrasing.

_____ **13.** The ability to participate in another person's feelings or ideas is called:

   A. empathy.

   B. redirection.

   C. restatement.

   D. counter-phrasing.

_____ **14.** Which of the following is false regarding dealing with a potentially violent patient?

   A. A person who is pacing or cannot sit still is likely to become violent.

   B. A person's posture is not an accurate means of assessing violence potential.

   C. Loud, obscene, or bizarre speech indicates emotional instability.

   D. When all interventions fail, law enforcement may need to be summoned.

_____ **15.** Factors to be considered before applying force to restrain a patient include all of the following EXCEPT:

   A. the type of abnormal behavior exhibited.

   B. the size, strength, and sex of the patient.

   C. approval from medical control.

   D. the type of restraint.

_____ **16.** Management of a suicide crisis includes:

   A. treatment of injuries, if necessary.

   B. support of the patient's ABCs as needed.

   C. emotional support.

   D. all of the above.

_____ **17.** Signs and symptoms of extreme stress include:

   A. lack of interest in sleep.

   B. lack of interest in food.

   C. hyperactivity.

   D. all of the above.

_____ **18.** Which of the following statements regarding dealing with death and dying is false?

   A. Dealing with your own feelings is not necessary when comforting others.

   B. Do not make false statements about the situation.

   C. Do whatever you can to meet the patient's medical needs.

   D. Consider the psychological needs of the patient and family.

_____ **19.** Because sexual assault creates an emotional crisis:

   A. the posttraumatic aspects of treatment are important.

   B. the physical aspects of treatment are important.

   C. the physiological aspects of treatment are important.

   D. the psychological aspects of treatment are important.

_____ **20.** Which of the following is false regarding dealing with an armed patient?

   A. If you are confronted by an armed person, immediately attempt to defend yourself.

   B. It is not your role to handle this situation unless you are a law enforcement officer.

   C. Do not proceed into an area where there may be an armed person without assistance from law enforcement.

   D. If you must wait for law enforcement, stay in your vehicle in a safe location.

True/False

If you believe the statement to be more true than false, write the letter "T" in the space provided. If you believe the statement to be more false than true, write the letter "F."

_____ **1.** In your role as an emergency medical responder, you should give psychological and emotional support to patients as well as emergency medical care.

_____ **2.** Sudden illness, injury, or death will almost always cause emotional upset or turmoil for those involved.

_____ **3.** When a person cannot cope with sudden or unexpected events, the person may act strange or even demonstrate dangerous behavior.

_____ **4.** As an EMR, you will rarely intervene in a situational crisis.

_____ **5.** Your interest in helping someone can be communicated by establishing eye contact.

_____ **6.** Even in serious situations, you can reassure a patient and still be honest by saying that everything possible is being done to help the patient.

_____ **7.** Standing above a patient with your hands on your hips assures the patient that you are a confident professional.

_____ **8.** Simple acts of kindness, such as offering a tissue or blanket, can often comfort a person who is emotionally upset and can sometimes lessen the severity of the crisis reaction.

_____ **9.** An appropriate sense of humor is important in emergency situations.

_____ **10.** A calm attitude on your part may help to calm a person who is in a crisis situation.

_____ **11.** If you have negative feelings about a patient, you should avoid caring for that patient.

_____ **12.** The best way to avoid violence against EMRs is prevention.

_____ **13.** Head injuries and shock may cause behavioral emergencies.

_____ **14.** High fevers and excess cold may cause behavioral emergencies.

_____ **15.** Psychotic behavior is characterized by defective or lost contact with reality.

_____ **16.** A state of emotional upset or turmoil caused by a sudden and disruptive event is called psychotic behavior.

_____ **17.** A person who is in emotional shock will not exhibit any of the physical signs of other types of shock.

_____ **18.** In a situational crisis, when a patient expresses denial, it is the responsibility of the EMR to quietly but firmly keep repeating the reality.

_____ **19.** During a situational crisis, a person begins screaming at you, calls you incompetent, and swears at you. You should immediately leave the scene and call your supervisor.

_____ **20.** Anger is difficult to handle objectively because it may seem to be directed at you personally.

_____ **21.** Treatment of a patient who is exhibiting abnormal behavior does not require the same steps of the patient assessment sequence as does treatment of other patients.

_____ **22.** If a patient is exhibiting abnormal behavior, the EMR should not try to communicate with him or her.

_____ **23.** Effective communication with a patient requires body language that exhibits empathy and interest.

_____ **24.** The best way to reassure patients is to tell them that everything is all right.

_____ **25.** Crisis intervention techniques include touching the patient.

_____ **26.** Crisis intervention techniques include good eye contact and a calm, steady voice.

_____ **27.** In crisis management, the most important step you can take is to talk with the person.

_____ **28.** A good way to reassure a patient and to show that you understand is simply to say, "I know what you mean" or "I know how you feel."

_____ **29.** Empathy can best be expressed by telling the patient that you know exactly how he or she feels.

_____ **30.** The technique of redirection may call for movement of the patient.

_____ **31.** Redirection is an attempt to alleviate the patient's concerns and bring attention back to the immediate situation.

_____ **32.** Trying to understand the emotional and psychological trauma that a patient experiences is using the technique of empathy.

_____ **33.** If the presence of too many emergency personnel at the scene is adding to a patient's anxiety, it is the responsibility of the EMR to ask them to move to another location.

_____ **34.** Crowds that may become hostile are the responsibility of law enforcement officers, not EMRs.

_____ **35.** An EMR will identify himself or herself to the patient and give reassurance that he or she is there to help.

_____ **36.** If you suspect abuse, your responsibility is to maintain safety for yourself and for the patient.

_____ **37.** Good communication skills for an EMR include the use of restatement and redirection.

_____ **38.** The tension phase is usually the shortest part of the abuse cycle.

_____ **39.** There should always be an escape route between you and the patient at scenes that may become dangerous.

_____ **40.** Your ability to use good interpersonal communication skills will help prevent many situations from becoming violent.

_____ **41.** If a patient who appears to be disturbed refuses to accept treatment, it may be necessary to provide care against the patient's will.

_____ **42.** Not all suicide attempts need to be taken seriously.

_____ **43.** Posttraumatic stress disorder is a severe form of anxiety.

_____ **44.** When treating a patient who was sexually assaulted, it is important to let them bathe and use the restroom.

_____ **45.** Coping with the death of others is a routine aspect of your job as an EMR.

_____ **46.** If you let stress build up without releasing it in healthy ways, it can begin to have negative effects on you and your performance.

_____ **47.** CISD teams may be helpful to rescuers who have been through an overwhelming or stressful event.

Crossword Puzzle

Use the clues in the column to complete the crossword puzzle.

Across

1. This phase of a situational crisis may follow denial or, in some cases, may occur instead of denial.

5. The best way to avoid violence at the scene of a behavioral emergency.

6. The third phase of the abuse cycle, when the abuser may make all sorts of promises, which are seldom kept.

8. One of the main causes of suicide in older people.

10. When communicating with the patient, try to position yourself so you are at the patient's _____.

Down

2. The second phase of the abuse cycle, when the abuser becomes enraged and loses control as well as the ability to think clearly.

3. If you are confronted by an armed person on scene, immediately attempt to _____.

4. Working alone or in _____ increases the risk of violence in the workplace.

7. A process developed by psychologists to help prevent excess stress and to relieve stress caused by critical incidents.

9. Loud, obscene, or bizarre _____ may indicate emotional instability.

Critical Thinking

Fill-in-the-Blank

Read each item carefully and then complete the statement by filling in the missing words.

1. Every emergency creates some sort of a(n) _____ _____ for the patient and for those close to the patient.

2. _____ is a normal human response to emotional overload or frustration.

3. _____ can help focus the patient's attention on the immediate situation.

4. Trying to put yourself in the patient's shoes is known as _____.

5. Many suicide attempts are really _____ _____ _____.

6. Performing simple _____ _____ may help reduce a patient's anxiety when there are many people around.

7. Abuse has been described as a(n) _____-part cycle.

8. Your most important assessment skill may be your ability to _____ with the patient.

9. There are _____ emotional phases to each situational crisis.

10. _____ and a sense of helplessness can often build to anger.

Short Answer

Complete this section with short written answers using the space provided.

1. List the five main factors that can cause behavioral changes.

_____

_____

2. What are some principles you should use when assessing patients with a behavioral problem?

_____

_____

3. What is the proper patient assessment sequence for a patient with a behavioral emergency?

_____

_____

4. When is it acceptable to provide care against the patient's will?

_____

_____

5. Name four factors that increase the risk of violence in the workplace.

_____

_____

6. What are the three types of death that an EMR may encounter?

_____

_____

7. List at least three signs and symptoms of extreme stress.

_____

_____

8. What is the purpose of CISD?

_____

_____

9. Provide a response to each of the following statements using the technique of restatement. In addition to rephrasing the statement to show that you understand, try to add some reassuring or encouraging words.

   A. From a woman who has been hit by a car: "I can't stay here! I have to go home and start dinner for the kids!"

   _____

   B. From the driver of the car that hit the woman: "I didn't mean to hit her! She just ran out all of a sudden! What if she dies?"

   _____

   C. From one of the woman's children, who was with her but not struck by the car: "I want my mommy! Let me go to my mommy!"

   _____

10. Provide a response to each of the statements in Question 9 using the technique of redirection.

   A. _____

   B. _____

   C. _____

You Make the Call

The following scenarios provide an opportunity to explore the concerns associated with patient management. Read the scenarios and answer the questions to the best of your ability.

1. When you arrive on the scene, you find a 24-year-old woman pacing the room and crying loudly. When you approach her, she pushes you away, saying, "I don't want your help; nobody can help me." She then turns her back to you and continues to pace. According to her friend, she and her boyfriend had a big fight, and he just left. What should you do?

_____

_____

_____

2. You respond to the scene of a suspected drug overdose. When you arrive on scene, you are greeted by a neighbor who tells you she found the patient in her closed garage, sitting in her car with the engine running. She said the patient was crying and stated, "I don't really want to die, but I just can't deal with this anymore." After you verify the engine is shut off and the garage doors are open, you approach the patient, a 36-year-old woman. How are you going to manage this patient?

_____

_____

_____

Environmental Emergencies

General Knowledge

Matching

Match each of the items in the left column to the appropriate definition in the right column.

_____ **1.** Drowning

_____ **2.** Frostbite

_____ **3.** Heat cramps

_____ **4.** Heat exhaustion

_____ **5.** Heatstroke

_____ **6.** Hypothermia

_____ **7.** Laryngospasm

_____ **8.** Submersion injury

A. Internal body temperature falls below 95°F (35°C)

B. Too much water and electrolyte loss due to heavy sweating after heat exposure

C. Suffocation because of submersion in water or other fluids

D. Injury resulting from being beneath the surface of water or another fluid

E. Body's mechanisms for heat release are overwhelmed due to a rapidly rising internal temperature

F. Muscle spasms that usually occur after vigorous exercise in hot weather

G. Spasm of vocal cords resulting in an inability to breathe

H. Freezing of the skin and deeper tissues

Multiple Choice

Read each item carefully and then select the one best response.

_____ **1.** Immediate emergency medical care for a patient who has heatstroke should consist of:

    A. calling for help.

    B. arranging for rapid transport to the hospital.

    C. giving the patient a drink of cool water and then treating for shock.

    D. maintaining the patient's ABCs, then lowering the body temperature as quickly as possible.

_____ **2.** Which of the following statements is true regarding the treatment of mild shock caused by heat exhaustion?

    A. Monitoring the patient's ABCs is usually not necessary.

    B. The patient should be soaked in cold water.

    C. The patient should be given a drink of cool water unless he or she is unconscious, nauseated, or vomiting.

    D. The patient's feet and legs should not be elevated.

_____ **3.** Which of the following signs and symptoms is associated with hypothermia?

    A. Agitation

    B. Sleepiness

    C. Bright red skin

    D. Elevated body temperature

_____ **4.** Your first step in caring for a patient with hypothermia should be to:

    A. treat the patient for shock.

    B. give the patient something to eat and drink.

    C. help the patient walk around to produce more body heat.

    D. move the patient to a warmer location and remove any wet clothing.

_____ **5.** A patient who is suffering from hypothermia may become unconscious at what body core temperature?

    A. 80° to 88°F (27° to 31°C)

    B. 89° to 92°F (32° to 33°C)

    C. 93° to 95°F (34° to 35°C)

    D. 95° to 97°F (35° to 36°C)

_____ **6.** The symptoms of dizziness, nausea, profuse sweating, weak pulse, and light-headedness indicate:

    A. heatstroke.

    B. heat exhaustion.

    C. hypothermia.

    D. none of the above.

_____ **7.** The symptoms of hot and red skin, loss of consciousness, and high body temperature are indications of:

    A. heatstroke.

    B. heat exhaustion.

    C. hypothermia.

    D. none of the above.

_____ **8.** Which of the following statements is false regarding frostbite?

    A. It may occur on the face.

    B. Wind speed may be a factor.

    C. Age, exhaustion, and hunger may increase susceptibility.

    D. It occurs only after an extended exposure to cold in an outdoor environment.

_____ **9.** If a person's body is not able to produce enough energy to keep its core temperature at a satisfactory level, the person has:

    A. hypothermia.

    B. superficial frostbite.

    C. deep frostbite.

    D. heat exhaustion.

_____ **10.** A patient's symptoms include shivering, sleepiness, and feeling cold. These symptoms indicate:

    A. deep frostbite.

    B. superficial frostbite.

    C. hypothermia.

    D. heat deprivation.

_____ **11.** Which of the following statements regarding drowning is false?

    A. Drowning is the second leading cause of injury and death among children 1 to 14 years.

    B. Alcohol consumption is not a contributing factor in drowning incidents involving teenagers.

    C. Young children can drown in liquids as shallow as 6 inches.

    D. The process of drowning progresses through several stages.

_____ **12.** When you encounter a person who has been submerged in cold water for an extended period of time:

    A. do not begin CPR until the core temperature rises to above 95°F (35°C).

    B. begin rescue breathing, but do not attempt CPR until an AED is available.

    C. CPR should be started and continued until the patient is delivered to an appropriate medical facility.

    D. CPR should be initiated if the submersion lasted less than 15 minutes.

_____ **13.** Which of the following statements is false regarding electrical injuries from a lightning strike?

    A. All patients should be transported to a medical facility.

    B. Lightning strikes can result in internal burns.

    C. Lightning strikes can cause cardiac irregularities or cardiac arrest.

    D. Cardiac problems are only seen within the first hour after the strike.

_____ **14.** Which of the following statements regarding the assessment of a patient with an environmental emergency is false?

    A. It is typically best to collect a medical history on the patient before you perform a secondary assessment.

    B. The patient is usually aware of the various aspects of his or her problems.

    C. You should review the dispatch information to help decide on possible treatment for the patient's problem.

    D. The SAMPLE history format will help collect the information you need to provide effective medical care.

_____ **15.** Which of the following is not a sign or symptom of a submersion injury?

    A. Diarrhea

    B. Vomiting

    C. Respiratory distress

    D. Coughing

True/False

If you believe the statement to be more true than false, write the letter "T" in the space provided. If you believe the statement to be more false than true, write the letter "F."

_____ **1.** The elderly and persons who are exhausted or hungry are more susceptible to frostbite.

_____ **2.** A person must be exposed to the cold for a long time to sustain frostbite injuries, even on very cold, windy days.

_____ **3.** In cases of frostbite, exposed body parts actually freeze.

_____ **4.** In the first stage of superficial frostbite, the exposed body part becomes pale white.

_____ **5.** If a person with frostbite has been out in the cold for hours, you should arrange for transport to the hospital rather than try to rewarm the affected body parts yourself.

_____ **6.** As an EMR, your emergency medical care of frostbite will consist of rewarming the affected body parts and treating the patient for signs of shock.

_____ **7.** Although you should never rub a frostbitten area with snow or ice, rubbing the area with your hands or a cloth is a good way to rewarm the area.

_____ **8.** The core body temperature of a person with hypothermia is lower than normal.

_____ **9.** Hypothermia occurs only in conditions of extreme cold.

_____ **10.** You should remove all wet clothing from a person who has hypothermia.

_____ **11.** Left untreated, hypothermia is serious but rarely fatal.

_____ **12.** If a patient who has hypothermia is conscious, you should give the patient something warm to drink.

_____ **13.** If at all possible, you should move a patient who has hypothermia to a warmer place.

_____ **14.** If a patient goes into cardiac arrest as a result of hypothermia, you should immediately begin CPR.

_____ **15.** A person with hypothermia who may have been considered dead for hours can be revived in the hospital.

_____ **16.** Heatstroke may cause brain damage or death.

_____ **17.** The most important step in treating heatstroke is rehydration.

_____ **18.** Frostbite and hypothermia may be encountered at any time of the year.

_____ **19.** Exercise, age, and medications may all be factors in heat-related illness.

_____ **20.** A patient showing indications of heat exhaustion should not be moved until ABCs are monitored and blood pressure is stabilized.

_____ **21.** A patient with deep frostbite should be transported to a medical facility for treatment.

_____ **22.** If a patient who appears to have hypothermia stops shivering, it is safe to assume that the patient has recovered and needs no treatment.

_____ **23.** CPR should be used on hypothermic patients even if there are no vital signs to indicate life.

_____ **24.** All patients who have sustained a submersion injury should be examined by a physician.

_____ **25.** The mammalian diving reflex increases the heart rate and metabolic rate while decreasing the body's demand for oxygen.

Crossword Puzzle

Use the clues in the column to complete the crossword puzzle.

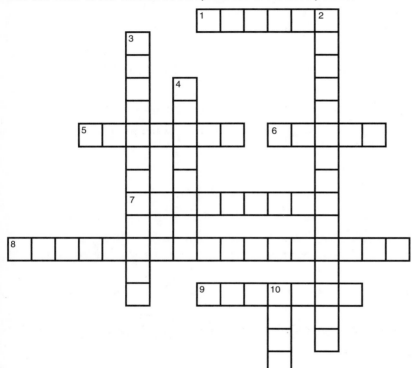

Across

1. Patients experiencing heat exhaustion usually have a(n) _____ body temperature.
5. The body parts most susceptible to frostbite are the face, ears, _____, and toes.
6. The initial stage in the process of drowning.
7. The body's attempt to produce more heat.
8. In this type of environmental emergency, the patient's mammalian diving reflex may be activated.
9. Fifty percent of the cases of infant drowning occur in this location.

Down

2. This type of injury can cause electrical burns and cardiac irregularities or arrest.
3. A submersion injury caused by small quantities of water reaching the larynx (voice box).
4. Heat cramps often occur after this activity, especially in hot weather.
10. Patients experiencing heatstroke usually have a(n) _____ body temperature.

Critical Thinking

Fill-in-the-Blank

Read each item carefully and then complete the statement by filling in the missing words.

1. Identify each of the following signs and symptoms associated with heat exhaustion or heatstroke by writing "HE," "HS," or both in the space provided.

   _____ **A.** Low blood pressure
   _____ **B.** Light-headedness or dizziness
   _____ **C.** High body temperature

	D. Profuse sweating
_____	**E.** Semiconsciousness or unconsciousness
_____	**F.** Flushed, dry skin
_____	**G.** Weak pulse
_____	**H.** Nausea

2. Drinking _____ _____ is an excellent treatment for patients experiencing heat exhaustion.

3. _____ is defined as suffocation because of submersion in water or other fluids.

4. There have been cases in which a person was submerged in cold water for over _____ _____ and was still successfully resuscitated.

5. For someone who is drowning, the feeling of panic produces a(n) _____ breathing pattern.

6. For children ages 5 to 14 years, most drownings occur in _____ and _____.

7. As the body temperature drops and hypothermia progresses, _____ stops.

8. Do not try to warm a frostbitten area by _____ it with your hands.

9. One way to help cool a patient is to place ice packs on the patient's _____.

10. In heatstroke, the patient's body temperature rises until it reaches a level at which _____ _____ occurs.

Fill-in-the-Table

Fill in the missing parts of the table.

Comparing Heat Exhaustion and Heatstroke	
Heat Exhaustion	**Heatstroke**
_____ body temperature	_____ body temperature
_____	_____ skin (usually)
_____ and _____ skin	_____ and _____ skin
Dizziness and _____	Semiconscious (or _____)

Short Answer

Complete this section with short written answers using the space provided.

1. Name the four body parts most susceptible to frostbite.

_____

_____

2. List the five common signs and symptoms of heat exhaustion.

_____

_____

3. Explain why older adults are more susceptible to heat and cold injuries.

_____

_____

4. What are the steps involved in the treatment of a patient with heatstroke?

_____

_____

You Make the Call

The following scenarios provide an opportunity to explore the concerns associated with patient management. Read the scenarios and answer the questions to the best of your ability.

1. You are at a family reunion at a local community park. You hear a cry for help down by the stream and find a young girl screaming that her brother fell in the stream and cannot swim. When you get near the stream, you see a young boy face down in the water. He is not moving. What should you do?

_____

_____

_____

2. You respond to a local church festival on a community service detail. Shortly after your arrival, you are summoned to one of the food stands for a man who is ill. When you arrive, you find a 62-year-old man with cold, sweaty skin, who complains of dizziness and nausea. The ambient temperature outside is 88°F (31°C), and it is much warmer inside the food stand. How should you treat this patient?

_____

_____

_____

Bleeding, Shock, and Soft-Tissue Injuries

General Knowledge

Matching

Match each of the items in the left column to the appropriate definition in the right column.

_____ 1. Abrasion   **A.** Injury that breaks the skin or mucous membrane

_____ 2. Avulsion   **B.** Soft-tissue damage occurs beneath the skin but there is no break in the skin surface

_____ 3. Bruise   **C.** Excessive bleeding

_____ 4. Closed wound   **D.** Two lower chambers of the heart

_____ 5. Cravat   **E.** Point where an injurious object passes out of the body

_____ 6. Exit wound   **F.** A piece of skin either torn off completely or left hanging as a flap

_____ 7. Full-thickness burns   **G.** Burns in which the outer layers of skin are burned

_____ 8. Hemorrhage   **H.** Results in inadequate delivery of blood to the organs of the body

_____ 9. Laceration   **I.** Burns that extend through the skin and into or beyond the underlying tissues

_____ 10. Open wound   **J.** Irregular cut or tear through the skin

_____ 11. Partial-thickness burns   **K.** Wound resulting from a bullet, knife, or any other pointed object

_____ 12. Puncture   **L.** Loss of skin due to a body part being scraped across a rough or hard surface

_____ 13. Shock   **M.** Triangular swathe of cloth

_____ 14. Thermal burns   **N.** Burns caused by heat

_____ 15. Ventricles   **O.** Injury caused by a blunt object striking the body and crushing the tissue beneath the skin

Multiple Choice

Read each item carefully and then select the one best response.

_____ 1. What is the most common cause of death in trauma patients?

     A. Internal bleeding

     B. External wounds

     C. Shock

     D. Cardiac arrest

_____ 2. Components of the circulatory system include all of the following EXCEPT:

     A. the pipes: arteries, veins, and capillaries.

     B. the fluid: blood cells and other blood components.

     C. the pressure wave: the pulse.

     D. the pump: the heart.

_____ 3. The lower chambers of the heart:

     A. are smaller than the upper chambers.

     B. do most of the actual pumping.

     C. are called atria.

     D. all of the above.

_____ **4.** The upper chambers of the heart:

    A. serve as reservoirs for blood.

    B. are called atria.

    C. are less muscular than the lower chambers.

    D. all of the above.

_____ **5.** The red blood cells:

    A. have a "search-and-destroy" function.

    B. carry oxygen and carbon dioxide.

    C. interact with one another to form blood clots.

    D. all of the above.

_____ **6.** The white blood cells:

    A. consume bacteria and viruses.

    B. interact with one another to form blood clots.

    C. serve as a transporting medium for other parts of the blood.

    D. all of the above.

_____ **7.** Which of the following statements regarding the pulse is incorrect?

    A. Taking a patient's pulse is the same as counting heartbeats.

    B. The pulse is the pressure wave generated by the pumping action of the heart.

    C. It does not reflect the heart rate.

    D. It is caused by the blood being pushed into the main arteries.

_____ **8.** Shock, or failure of the circulatory system, is NOT caused by:

    A. pressure loss.

    B. pipe failure.

    C. fluid loss.

    D. pump failure.

_____ **9.** If the heart is incapable of pumping enough blood to supply the needs of the body:

    A. blood can back up in the vessels of the lungs, causing congestive heart failure.

    B. cardiogenic shock may occur.

    C. the patient may have had a heart attack.

    D. all of the above.

_____ **10.** Shock, as a result of capillary expansion, includes all of the following EXCEPT:

    A. shock related to respiratory failure.

    B. shock induced by fainting.

    C. anaphylactic shock.

    D. spinal shock.

_____ **11.** Psychogenic shock:

    A. is the least serious type of shock, caused by pipe failure.

    B. is known as fainting.

    C. will correct itself if the patient is placed in a horizontal position.

    D. all of the above.

_____ **12.** Anaphylactic shock:

    A. is caused by fluid loss.

    B. is usually caused by hemorrhage.

    C. may be accompanied by itching, rash, hives, or swelling of the face or tongue.

    D. all of the above.

_____ **13.** Shock caused by a temporary reduction in blood supply to the brain is called:
  A. anaphylactic shock.
  B. psychogenic shock.
  C. cardiogenic shock.
  D. all of the above.

_____ **14.** Shock caused by an allergic reaction to food, medicine, or insect stings is called:
  A. anaphylactic shock.
  B. psychogenic shock.
  C. cardiogenic shock.
  D. all of the above.

_____ **15.** Signs and symptoms of shock may include all of the following EXCEPT:
  A. nausea and vomiting.
  B. confusion, restlessness, or anxiety.
  C. thirst.
  D. decreased capillary refill time.

_____ **16.** Which of the following is false regarding shock?
  A. You should not allow a shock patient to stand.
  B. Raise the patient's legs 12" to 18" off the floor.
  C. If the patient is having chest pain and no spinal injury is suspected, place the patient in a sitting or semireclining position.
  D. Assess the patient's ABCs at least every 5 minutes.

_____ **17.** General treatment for shock includes:
  A. giving the patient sips of water or other fluids.
  B. getting the patient to walk as soon as possible.
  C. maintaining the patient's ABCs.
  D. all of the above.

_____ **18.** Positioning a patient who shows signs of shock may include:
  A. placing a blanket under the patient.
  B. elevating the patient's legs.
  C. placing the patient flat on his or her back.
  D. all of the above.

_____ **19.** The EMR can treat a patient who exhibits signs and symptoms of shock by doing all of the following EXCEPT:
  A. treating the cause of shock.
  B. starting an IV line.
  C. maintaining the patient's ABCs.
  D. maintaining the body temperature of the patient.

_____ **20.** Upon arrival of ALS units, a patient who is in shock may be treated with:
  A. a pneumatic antishock garment (PASG).
  B. IV fluids.
  C. oxygen.
  D. all of the above.

_____ **21.** Patients experiencing shock caused by pump failure may present with:
  A. a rapid, weak pulse.
  B. cold, clammy, sweaty, and pale skin.
  C. rapid, shallow respirations.
  D. all of the above.

_____ **22.** Which of the following is NOT part of the treatment of a gunshot wound?

  A. Begin CPR if the patient's heart stops within 5 minutes of the injury.

  B. Examine the patient thoroughly to be sure you have discovered all entrance and exit wounds.

  C. Arrange for prompt transport of the patient.

  D. Maintain the patient's body temperature.

_____ **23.** If an object is impaled in the patient:

  A. remove the object and apply a stabilizing dressing.

  B. remove the object and apply a regular dressing.

  C. leave the object in place, apply a stabilizing dressing, and arrange for transport.

  D. remove the object, apply a stabilizing dressing, and arrange for transport.

_____ **24.** An amputated body part should be:

  A. located and placed in a clean plastic bag.

  B. kept cold.

  C. taken with the patient to the hospital.

  D. all of the above.

_____ **25.** Signs and symptoms of internal blood loss include all of the following EXCEPT:

  A. rectal and/or vaginal bleeding.

  B. coughing or vomiting of blood.

  C. abdominal tenderness, rigidity, or distention.

  D. bleeding from a wound.

_____ **26.** Treatment of shock caused by external blood loss includes which of the following steps?

  A. Providing glucose

  B. Elevating the head

  C. Applying direct pressure to the wound

  D. All of the above

_____ **27.** External bleeding can be controlled by:

  A. application of direct pressure.

  B. elevation of the body part.

  C. application of pressure at the pressure point.

  D. all of the above.

_____ **28.** In applying femoral pressure, you should:

  A. kneel on the same side as the injury.

  B. position the patient on his or her side.

  C. be facing the patient's head.

  D. all of the above.

_____ **29.** Which of the following is false regarding a closed wound?

  A. It is a bruise or contusion.

  B. It is an injury of the soft tissue beneath the skin.

  C. It causes discoloration and swelling.

  D. It includes abrasions and lacerations.

_____ **30.** An abrasion:

  A. is caused by a sharp object that penetrates the skin.

  B. is the tearing away of body tissue.

  C. may be called road rash or a rug burn.

  D. all of the above.

_____ **31.** Avulsion:

    A. is the most common type of open wound.

    B. is the tearing away of body tissue.

    C. may be caused by a sharp object penetrating the skin.

    D. all of the above.

_____ **32.** An occlusive dressing:

    A. is used for open chest wounds.

    B. is used to maintain air pressure in the lungs.

    C. can be plastic wrap or aluminum foil.

    D. all of the above.

_____ **33.** A burn that damages all layers of the skin:

    A. may not be accompanied by pain.

    B. may make the patient susceptible to shock and infection.

    C. is called a full-thickness or third-degree burn.

    D. all of the above.

_____ **34.** A respiratory burn:

    A. may cause breathing problems.

    B. will not cause any pain.

    C. will be visible immediately.

    D. all of the above.

_____ **35.** You are called to the scene where a 16-year-old boy has been beaten severely and is unresponsive. You should first feel for a pulse at which artery?

    A. Brachial

    B. Radial

    C. Carotid

    D. Temporal

_____ **36.** After a patient has fainted and has been placed in the correct position, you should maintain the patient's ABCs and then:

    A. shout at and shake the patient until he or she becomes responsive.

    B. treat the cause of shock, if possible.

    C. call for help and keep the patient extra warm.

    D. call for help and watch for signs of responsiveness so you can immediately lower the patient's legs.

_____ **37.** Which of the following signs can develop quickly in a person who is in anaphylactic shock?

    A. Rash

    B. Pale skin

    C. Strong pulse

    D. High blood pressure

_____ **38.** After placing the patient in the correct position, what is the first thing you should do for a patient who is in shock?

    A. Give the patient some water to drink.

    B. Give the patient something to eat.

    C. Maintain the patient's ABCs.

    D. Begin one-rescuer CPR.

_____ 39. A small boy has severe bleeding from a cut on the back of his head. No brain tissue or bone chips are visible. He is sitting on the ground, sobbing and clinging to his mother. His mother tells you he was hit by a swing and begs you to do something before he "bleeds to death." The first step in providing care is to:

    A. reassure the mother that the boy will be fine.

    B. treat the boy immediately for shock from blood loss.

    C. apply direct pressure to the wound and then reassure the boy and his mother that you are trying to help.

    D. cover the wound and then bandage it loosely in case of skull fracture.

_____ 40. You are called to a softball field where a young man has a scalp laceration after he is hit in the head with a ball. You check the man's airway and breathing and treat the wound. No brain tissue or bone chips are showing. You should next check for changes in:

    A. pulse.

    B. body temperature.

    C. blood pressure.

    D. level of consciousness.

_____ 41. Although a burn patient may have severe pain, the real danger of burns that damage or destroy the skin is the loss of:

    A. nerve endings that signal further injuries.

    B. dehydration caused by the heat of the burns.

    C. the skin's ability to prevent infection-causing bacteria from entering the body and essential fluids from seeping out.

    D. the skin's ability to regulate body temperature.

_____ 42. Thermal burns, if still warm, should be immediately cooled with:

    A. butter.

    B. grease.

    C. cold water.

    D. burn ointment.

_____ 43. A man whose car battery exploded in his face is screaming and holding his hands over his eyes when you arrive. You grab a nearby garden hose to flush his eyes, but he will not remove his hands from his face. After you flush the man's eyes, you should:

    A. arrange for rapid transport to the hospital.

    B. allow the man to put his hands back over his eyes.

    C. tell the man to keep his hands away from his eyes and cover him with a burn sheet.

    D. cover his eyes with gauze bandages and arrange for prompt transport to an appropriate medical facility.

_____ 44. Pressure points should be used for extremity wounds in all of the following situations EXCEPT:

    A. if you are not permitted to use a tourniquet.

    B. after bleeding has stopped from application of direct pressure.

    C. if direct pressure does not control bleeding.

    D. if elevation does not control bleeding.

True/False

If you believe the statement to be more true than false, write the letter "T" in the space provided. If you believe the statement to be more false than true, write the letter "F."

_____ 1. When approaching a patient who may have sustained a soft-tissue injury, the EMR must remember to take appropriate standard precautions.

_____ 2. The heart is divided into two upper chambers, called ventricles, and two lower chambers, called atria.

_____ 3. The arteries return the blood to the heart and lungs, where it gives off carbon dioxide and absorbs oxygen.

_____ 4. The capillaries are the smallest of the blood vessels.

_____ 5. If a patient is in shock, the carotid pulse may be impossible to find, and it will be necessary to find the radial pulse instead.

_____ 6. The carotid pulse can be located and checked more easily than the radial pulse in a patient who is in shock.

_____   **7.** A state of collapse of the cardiovascular system that results in inadequate delivery of blood to the organs is known as shock.

_____   **8.** Anaphylactic shock may develop very quickly and, without rapid treatment, death may occur.

_____   **9.** Unchecked external or internal bleeding may cause shock and death.

_____   **10.** Skin color and condition are important factors in detecting shock in a patient.

_____   **11.** General treatment of shock should include proper positioning of the patient.

_____   **12.** A patient who has shown signs and symptoms of shock should have his or her ABCs checked every minute.

_____   **13.** EMRs may be able to treat the cause of shock if it is external bleeding.

_____   **14.** Treatment of a patient with anaphylactic shock includes prompt ambulance transport to an appropriate medical facility.

_____   **15.** Puncture wounds are caused by blunt objects that penetrate the skin.

_____   **16.** Not all wounds require bandaging.

_____   **17.** Excessive bleeding is the most common cause of shock.

_____   **18.** All eye injuries are potentially serious and require medical evaluation.

_____   **19.** The femoral artery pressure point is easier to locate and squeeze than the brachial artery.

_____   **20.** Use of tourniquets is only indicated in cases where bleeding cannot be controlled by direct pressure or elevation.

_____   **21.** An object that causes a puncture wound and remains sticking out of the skin is called an impaled object.

_____   **22.** Lacerations, a type of open wound, range in severity from minor to life threatening.

_____   **23.** Most bleeding from the scalp and face can be controlled by applying direct manual pressure.

_____   **24.** All neck injuries are considered serious because of the proximity of the trachea, the esophagus, large arteries, veins, muscles, vertebrae, and the spinal cord.

_____   **25.** If an abdominal wound causes the intestines to protrude from the abdomen, the intestines should be gently pushed into the opening before covering with a sterile dressing.

_____   **26.** A rapid, weak pulse is a common sign of shock.

_____   **27.** Nausea, vomiting, and thirst are not common signs of shock.

_____   **28.** Once you have placed a patient with a nosebleed in the correct position, you should pinch the nostrils together for at least 5 minutes.

_____   **29.** An occlusive dressing allows air to pass through it.

_____   **30.** Legs and arms with a significant amount of swelling or bruising should be splinted in case of an underlying fracture.

_____   **31.** Visible external electrical burns should be covered with a dry, sterile dressing.

_____   **32.** If a downed power line is sitting on the hood of a car and the people inside seem uninjured, you should tell them to leave the car.

_____   **33.** A person who is subjected to a strong electrical current can have severe internal damage.

_____   **34.** Injuries in multisystem trauma can occur in one part of the body but involve different body systems.

_____   **35.** When flushing an eye, flush from the nose side toward the outside to avoid flushing the object into the other eye.

_____   **36.** You should use tourniquets only if you have completed proper instruction and have approval from your medical director.

_____   **37.** Elevation, in conjunction with direct pressure, typically is not enough to stop severe bleeding.

Labeling

Label the following diagrams with the correct terms.

1. Parts of the Heart

A. _____

B. _____

C. _____

D. _____

E. _____

F. _____

G. _____

H. _____

I. _____

J. _____

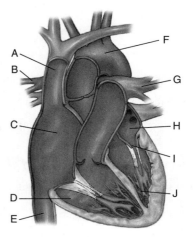

2. Types of External Bleeding

A. _____

B. _____

C. _____

A

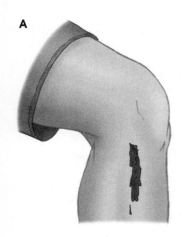

B

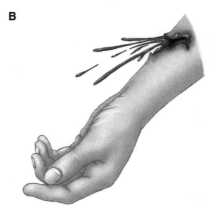

C

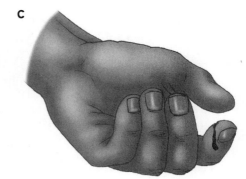

3. Types of Wounds

A. _____

B. _____

C. _____

D. _____

A
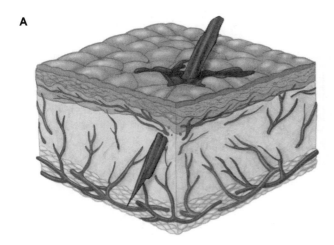

B
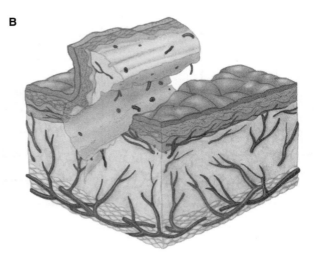

C
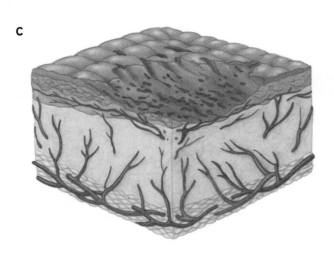

D
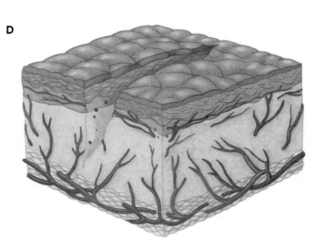

Crossword Puzzle

Use the clues in the column to complete the crossword puzzle.

Across

4. The _____ pressure point is located in the arm between the elbow and the shoulder; also used in taking blood pressure and for checking the pulse in infants.

7. Point where an injurious object such as a bullet enters the body.

9. A serious type of bleeding from an artery in which blood frequently pulses or spurts from an open wound.

11. Fluids other than blood or blood products infused into the vascular system to maintain an adequate circulatory blood volume.

12. Heart disease characterized by breathlessness, fluid retention in the lungs, and generalized swelling of the body.

13. Object placed directly on a wound to control bleeding and prevent further contamination.

14. A type of burn caused by contact with high- or low-voltage electricity; these burns have an entrance and an exit wound.

15. A type of shock commonly known as fainting; caused by a temporary reduction in blood supply to the brain.

Down

1. A severe type of shock caused by an allergic reaction to food, medicine, or insect stings.

2. Salt water.

3. A type of shock resulting from inadequate functioning of the heart.

5. An abrasion caused by sliding on pavement. Usually seen after motorcycle or bicycle accidents.

6. The _____ pressure point is located in the groin, where the femoral artery is close to the skin.

8. A means of immobilizing an injured part by using a rigid or soft support.

10. An acute viral infection of the central nervous system transmitted by the bite of an infected animal.

Critical Thinking

Fill-in-the-Blank

Read each item carefully and then complete the statement by filling in the missing words.

1. Using the rule of nines, calculate the percentage of the body that would be burned in each scenario for an adult patient.

   _____ **A.** Both legs

   _____ **B.** The groin, the front of the trunk, and the head

   _____ **C.** One half of the front of the trunk and one arm

   _____ **D.** The backs of both arms and the back

   _____ **E.** The fronts of both legs and the groin

2. Identify each sign or characteristic as associated with first-, second-, or third-degree burns by placing the numbers 1, 2, and/or 3 in the space provided.

_____   **A.** May not require medical treatment

_____   **B.** All layers of skin damaged

_____   **C.** Moderate to severe pain

_____   **D.** Loss of large quantities of body fluids

_____   **E.** Reddened skin

_____   **F.** Pain sometimes absent

_____   **G.** Minor to moderate pain

_____   **H.** Presence of blisters

_____   **I.** Deepest layers of skin not damaged

_____   **J.** Greatest risk of shock and infection

3. The use of _____ is indicated only in situations where extremity bleeding cannot be controlled by direct pressure or elevation.

4. If you get blood on your hands, _____ it off as soon as possible with _____ and _____.

5. Most deaths from gunshot wounds result from _____ blood loss.

6. If an entire body part is torn away, the wound is called a(n) _____ amputation.

7. It is important to stop bleeding as quickly as possible using the _____ dressing available.

8. A(n) _____ is an object placed directly on a wound to control bleeding and prevent further contamination.

9. Two types of bandages commonly used in the field are _____ _____ and _____ _____.

10. Once you have completed applying the bandage, _____ it so that it cannot _____.

11. Severe scalp lacerations may be associated with _____ _____ or even _____ _____.

12. A nosebleed with no apparent cause is called a(n) _____ nosebleed.

13. If the patient is vomiting blood, it may be an indication of bleeding from the _____ or _____.

14. Injury to the genitals can often result in severe _____.

15. Some gunshot wounds are easy to miss unless you perform a thorough _____ _____.

16. All bites carry a high risk of causing _____.

17. If blisters are present with a burn, be very careful not to _____ the blisters.

18. When dealing with a chemical burn, you should _____ _____ any dry chemical on the patient's clothes or skin.

19. Chemical burns to the eyes can cause extreme _____ and severe _____.

20. Electricity causes major _____ damage, rather than _____ damage.

Short Answer

Complete this section with short written answers using the space provided.

1. Name the three primary parts of the circulatory system.

_____

_____

2. Name the three primary causes of shock.

_____

_____

3. Name three things you could use for an occlusive dressing.

_____

_____

4. What are the three classifications of burns?

_____

_____

5. What should you use to cover the affected area after a thermal burn has cooled?

_____

_____

6. Name three signs or symptoms of respiratory burns.

_____

_____

7. What are the steps for the general treatment of shock?

_____

_____

8. What are the steps for treating an open abdominal wound?

_____

_____

9. List the four major principles of open wound treatment.

_____

_____

You Make the Call

The following scenarios provide an opportunity to explore the concerns associated with patient management. Read the scenarios and answer the questions to the best of your ability.

1. When you arrive at the scene, you find that your patient is a 6-year-old girl who was preparing breakfast to surprise her mother. She started the water boiling and when she attempted to pour it into a mug, the pan slipped and the boiling water burned her abdomen, the lower part of her left arm, and the fronts of both legs. Most of the burn area is covered with large blisters. Some of the blisters are intact, and others are broken with the skin peeling. What should you do?

_____

_____

_____

2. You are dispatched to a local machine shop for the report of a man with an injured arm. You are on the scene in less than 1 minute because you are one block away. As you arrive, you are told that the patient got his arm caught in a lathe, and he has a severe laceration and damage to his lower arm. Upon examination, you note blood spurting from the patient's lower arm. What should you do?

_____

_____

_____

Skills

Skill Drills

Test your knowledge of this skill by filling in the correct words in the photo caption.

Skill Drill 13-1: Controlling Bleeding With a Tourniquet

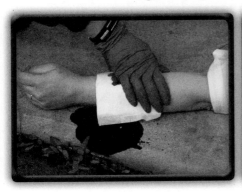 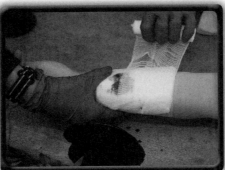 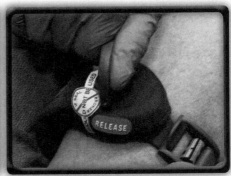

1. Apply _____ _____ with a sterile dressing.

2. Apply a _____ dressing.

3. If bleeding continues or recurs, apply a tourniquet _____ the level of bleeding.

Injuries to Muscles and Bones

General Knowledge

Matching

Match each of the items in the left column to the appropriate definition in the right column.

_____ **1.** Mechanism of injury

_____ **2.** Closed fracture

_____ **3.** Sprain

_____ **4.** Dislocation

_____ **5.** Paralysis

_____ **6.** Joint

_____ **7.** Trauma

_____ **8.** Seizures

_____ **9.** Osteoporosis

_____ **10.** Cerebrospinal fluid

A. Sudden episodes of uncontrolled electrical activity in the brain

B. The place where two bones come in contact with each other

C. The means by which a traumatic injury occurs

D. Joint injury in which the joint is partially or temporarily dislocated and supporting ligaments are either stretched or torn

E. Wound or injury, either physical or psychological

F. Fracture in which the overlying skin has not been damaged

G. Clear, watery, straw-colored fluid that fills the space between the brain and spinal chord

H. Disruption of a joint so that the bone ends are no longer in alignment

I. Abnormal brittleness of the bones in older people

J. Inability of a conscious person to move voluntarily

Multiple Choice

Read each item carefully and then select the one best response.

_____ **1.** Muscles of the body may be called:

    A. voluntary.

    B. involuntary.

    C. cardiac.

    D. all of the above.

_____ **2.** Muscles that can be contracted and relaxed by a person at will are called:

    A. voluntary.

    B. involuntary.

    C. cardiac.

    D. all of the above.

_____ **3.** Muscles that are found in the inside of the digestive tract and other internal organs are called:

    A. voluntary.

    B. involuntary.

    C. cardiac.

    D. all of the above.

_____ **4.** The mechanism of injury refers to:

    A. how to move an injured patient.

    B. whether a patient can move an injured limb.

    C. the means by which an injury has occurred.

    D. the type of transport needed for injuries.

_____ **5.** Musculoskeletal injuries may be caused by all of the following EXCEPT:

    A. direct force.

    B. oblique force.

    C. twisting force.

    D. indirect force.

_____ **6.** Which of the following does NOT describe musculoskeletal injuries?

    A. Fractures, dislocations, and sprains

    B. Closed and open fractures

    C. Warm and pink

    D. Painful, swollen, deformed extremity

_____ **7.** An injury that causes tears of the ligaments and separation of the bone ends is a(n):

    A. open fracture.

    B. sprain.

    C. dislocation.

    D. closed fracture.

_____ **8.** An injury in which a joint is partially dislocated and there is excessive stretching of supporting ligaments is called a(n):

    A. open fracture.

    B. sprain.

    C. dislocation.

    D. closed fracture.

_____ **9.** During examination of an injured limb, the EMR's best indicator of an underlying fracture, dislocation, or sprain is:

    A. an open wound.

    B. bruising.

    C. tenderness.

    D. swelling.

_____ **10.** Signs that indicate an injury to a limb may include all of the following EXCEPT:

    A. ability to bear weight.

    B. swelling or bruising.

    C. tenderness or pain with motion.

    D. deformity.

_____ **11.** Use of the capillary refill test:

    A. will indicate a circulation problem.

    B. takes 2 to 3 minutes.

    C. gives an accurate indication under all circumstances.

    D. all of the above.

_____ **12.** General principles of splinting limb injuries include which of the following?

    A. Do not splint joints unless injury is visible.

    B. Leave clothing in place.

    C. Pad all rigid splints.

    D. All of the above.

_____ **13.** Splints made from wood, aluminum, or plastic are called:

    A. rigid splints.

    B. traction splints.

    C. soft splints.

    D. commercial splints.

_____ **14.** A clear plastic, inflatable splint is a type of:

    A. rigid splint.

    B. traction splint.

    C. soft splint.

    D. all of the above.

_____ **15.** A triangular bandage or similar material tied around the neck to support the weight of an injured upper extremity is called a(n):

    A. improvised splint.

    B. sling.

    C. traction sling.

    D. rigid splint.

_____ **16.** Head injuries may cause:

    A. bleeding and/or swelling within the skull.

    B. seepage of CSF.

    C. injury to the spine.

    D. all of the above.

_____ **17.** What is the first step for an EMR to take if there are signs or symptoms of head injury?

    A. Check and maintain the airway.

    B. Call for additional help.

    C. Immobilize the head and stabilize the neck.

    D. Check circulation and for bleeding.

_____ **18.** When facial injuries are present:

    A. place the patient in the recovery position.

    B. bandage the entire head and face.

    C. stabilize the head in a neutral position.

    D. all of the above.

_____ **19.** Signs and symptoms of a spinal cord injury include all of the following EXCEPT:

    A. tenderness over any point on the spine or neck.

    B. increased bowel or bladder control.

    C. laceration, bruise, or other sign of injury to the head, neck, or spine.

    D. tingling or burning sensation in any part of the body below the neck.

_____ **20.** If a patient with injuries to the chest exhibits a reversed movement of the chest during breathing:

    A. he or she may need oxygen.

    B. suspect flail chest.

    C. place a pillow on the patient's chest.

    D. all of the above.

_____ **21.** One way a dislocation differs from a sprain is that in a dislocation:

    A. fewer nerves are damaged.

    B. there is less pain.

    C. the supporting ligaments are torn from the joint.

    D. the bones always realign into their natural position in the joint.

_____ **22.** An injury in which the bone is broken but the skin remains intact is called a(n):

    A. bruise.

    B. contusion.

    C. closed fracture.

    D. open fracture.

_____ **23.** Which of the following statements best describes an open fracture?

    A. The ends of the bones at the break are aligned but are more than an inch apart.

    B. The risk of infection is high because dirt and bacteria often enter the wound.

    C. Bleeding is minimal because the bone end causes a puncture wound.

    D. To break the bone, a bullet or some sharp object must have broken the skin.

_____ **24.** To determine if a patient has adequate circulation in an injured arm, you should check the _____ pulse.

    A. carotid

    B. radial

    C. tibial

    D. femoral

_____ **25.** Emergency care of a patient who has no pulse or capillary refill in an injured limb should be to:

    A. encourage the patient to move the limb.

    B. briskly rub the limb to stimulate circulation.

    C. warm the limb to stimulate circulation.

    D. arrange for immediate transport to a hospital.

_____ **26.** A man who shows no sign of injury in his arm is unable to make a fist. He has most likely injured what structures in the arm?

    A. Nerves

    B. Muscles

    C. Bones

    D. Tendons and ligaments

_____ **27.** To test for sensation in an injured arm, you should touch the tips of the _____ fingers.

    A. index and middle

    B. index and little

    C. middle and little

    D. middle and ring

_____ **28.** To test for sensation in an injured leg, you should touch the tip of the big toe and the:

    A. heel.

    B. arch of the foot.

    C. top of the foot.

    D. side of the little toe.

_____ **29.** You should always inflate a soft splint with:

    A. water.

    B. your mouth (breath).

    C. an air pump.

    D. an air cylinder.

_____ **30.** Most splinting operations require two people; the first applies the splint, and the second:

    A. inflates the splint.

    B. distracts the patient.

    C. stabilizes and supports the injured limb.

    D. makes sure the splint is applied properly.

_____ **31.** Emergency care of a patient who has a broken thighbone should include placing the patient in a comfortable position and:

    A. elevating the injured leg.

    B. bending the injured leg at the knee.

    C. treating the patient for shock.

    D. applying ice or cold compresses to the leg.

_____ **32.** You are in a remote rural area where a fire is burning near some farm equipment. You need to move a patient with a fractured thighbone, but EMTs will not arrive for another 10 minutes. The best way to prevent additional injury would be to:

    A. wait for the EMTs to arrive.

    B. try to put the fire out.

    C. leave the patient and find help.

    D. secure the injured leg to the uninjured leg and then move the patient.

_____ **33.** When responding to motor vehicle crashes with broken glass or other sharp objects:

    A. you should be more concerned about the patient than your safety.

    B. latex gloves will provide optimal protection.

    C. it is wise to wear heavy rescue gloves that provide protection from sharp objects.

    D. all of the above.

_____ **34.** Which of the following is not part of the treatment of hand, wrist, and finger injuries?

    A. Place one or two soft roller dressings on the back of the patient's hand.

    B. Cover all wounds with a dry, sterile dressing.

    C. Place the injured hand or wrist into a position of function.

    D. Apply a splint to hold the wrist, hand, and fingers in the position of function, and secure the splint with a soft roller bandage.

_____ **35.** Common causes of spinal cord injuries include all of the following EXCEPT:

    A. falls less than three times the patient's height.

    B. athletic collisions.

    C. hangings.

    D. diving injuries.

_____ **36.** Which of the following is false regarding the treatment of penetrating chest wounds?

    A. Quickly seal an open chest wound with a material that will prevent more air from entering the chest cavity.

    B. If a knife or other object is impaled in the chest, remove it immediately.

    C. Any chest injury that results in air leakage and bleeding requires prompt attention.

    D. A conscious patient with chest trauma may demand to be placed in a sitting position to ease breathing.

True/False

If you believe the statement to be more true than false, write the letter "T" in the space provided. If you believe the statement to be more false than true, write the letter "F."

_____ **1.** The skeletal system is divided into seven areas.

_____ **2.** The 12 sets of ribs provide protection for the heart and other organs and are attached to the spine and sternum.

_____ **3.** Each of the essential organs of the body is encased in a protective bony structure.

_____ **4.** Red blood cells are manufactured within the spaces inside the bone.

_____ **5.** In a closed fracture, the end of the broken bone will be visible through the broken skin.

_____ **6.** A thorough inspection and hands-on examination of an injured limb will not incorporate any information given by the patient verbally.

_____ **7.** The pulse of an injured limb should be checked at a point distal to the injury.

_____ **8.** The absence of a pulse or capillary refill in an injured limb indicates that the patient has been exposed to cold temperatures.

_____ **9.** Any open wound, deformity, swelling, or bruising of a limb should be considered evidence of a possible limb injury.

_____ **10.** Splinting of a limb injury is required only if the patient is unable to move it.

_____ **11.** Splinting prevents closed fractures from becoming open fractures during movement or transport.

_____ **12.** In a limb injury, notation of the pulse and sensation is not needed as long as the limb is splinted.

_____ **13.** An inflatable, clear plastic splint is inflated most easily and most effectively with a pump.

_____ **14.** Triangular bandages can effectively be used to immobilize and treat injuries to the shoulders.

_____ **15.** Hip fractures are breaks in the hip joint, only occurring as a result of high-energy trauma.

_____ **16.** A patient suspected of a hip fracture should be transported on a long backboard with splinting that uses pillows or blankets.

_____ **17.** Securing the two lower extremities together will allow for quick removal of a thigh-injury patient from a dangerous environment.

_____ **18.** Spinal injury and head injury are usually not closely related.

_____ **19.** During a motor vehicle crash, brain injury is often caused by the brain striking the inside of the skull.

_____ **20.** The primary danger in severe facial injuries is obstruction of the airway.

_____ **21.** Any facial injuries resulting in profuse bleeding require treatment for life-threatening injuries.

_____ **22.** Abdominal breathing is a sign or symptom that may indicate spinal injury.

_____ **23.** If spinal injury is suspected and there are breathing problems, the head tilt–chin lift technique should be used to open the airway.

_____ **24.** A long or short backboard and rigid collar are used to splint the cervical spine.

_____ **25.** Part of your visual examination should include comparing the injured limb with the opposite, uninjured limb.

_____ **26.** Even if there are no signs of injury after a thorough visual examination of a limb, you should examine the limb by feeling it with your hands.

_____ **27.** Every part of a limb should be squeezed gently but firmly during a hands-on examination.

_____ **28.** You should never ask a patient to move the limb after your visual and hands-on examination.

_____ **29.** All limbs with open wounds should be splinted before the open wound is covered.

_____ **30.** The only reason injured limbs are splinted in the field is to prevent further damage from occurring during transport.

_____ **31.** You may move the limb as much as you want when applying a splint to ensure that the splint is applied correctly.

_____ **32.** Hip dislocations are extremely painful, especially when any movement is attempted.

_____ **33.** A patient who has a fracture of the right hip will appear to have a shorter right leg.

_____ **34.** The most definite sign of a pelvic fracture is tenderness when you use both of your hands to firmly compress the patient's pelvis.

_____ **35.** You should quickly treat an open chest wound with an occlusive dressing.

_____ **36.** As you examine and treat patients with musculoskeletal injuries, you need to practice standard precautions.

_____ **37.** Patients with rib fractures should be splinted with pillows; however, oxygen therapy is generally not required.

Labeling

Label the following diagrams with the correct terms.

1. The Human Skeleton

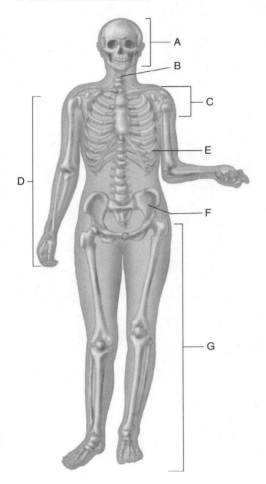

A. _____

B. _____

C. _____

D. _____

E. _____

F. _____

G. _____

2. Sections of the Spine

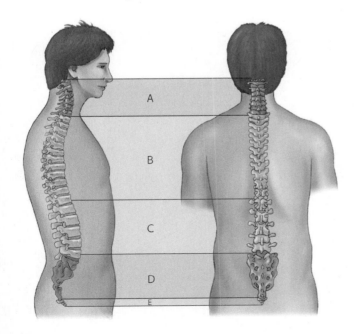

A. _____

B. _____

C. _____

D. _____

E. _____

3. Types of Muscle

A. _____

B. _____

C. _____

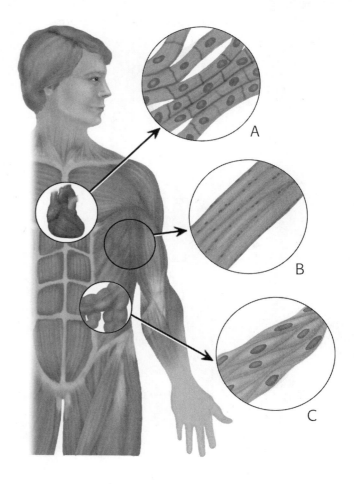

Crossword Puzzle

Use the clues in the column to complete the crossword puzzle.

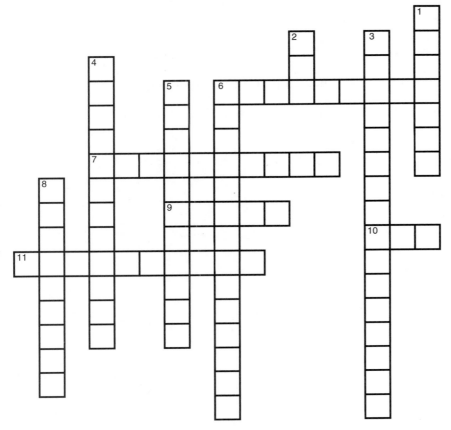

Across

6. The upper portion of the lower extremity; from the hip joint to the knee.

7. A chest injury in which three or more ribs are broken in two or more places, resulting in the injured part of the chest moving in the opposite direction from the rest of the chest.

9. A bandage or material that helps to support the weight of an injured upper extremity.

10. The upper portion of the upper extremity; from the shoulder to the elbow.

11. A splint made from supple material that provides gentle support.

Down

1. The lower portion of the upper extremity; from the elbow to the wrist.

2. The lower portion of the lower extremity; from the knee to the foot.

3. Injury where there is bleeding and/or swelling within the skull.

4. Any fracture in which the overlying skin has been damaged.

5. A splint made from firm materials such as wood, aluminum, or plastic.

6. A splint that holds a lower extremity fracture in alignment by applying a constant, steady pull on the extremity.

8. _____ breathing uses only the diaphragm.

Critical Thinking

Fill-in-the-Blank

Read each item carefully and then complete the statement by filling in the missing words.

1. Splinting of the cervical spine is accomplished with a(n) _____ _____ and a long or short spine board or backboard.

2. The primary danger in severe facial injuries is _____ of the airway.

3. How injuries occur is known as the _____ of injury.

4. A(n) _____ is a disruption that tears the supporting ligaments of the joint.

5. One sign of a head injury, known as _____ sign, is a bruise behind one or both ears.

6. A spinal cord injury may paralyze respiratory muscles and cause the patient to breathe using only the diaphragm, which is known as _____ breathing.

7. Fracture of three or more ribs in at least two places causes a condition known as _____ chest.

8. _____ is the abnormal brittleness of the bones in older people caused by loss of calcium.

9. For a patient with a spinal cord injury, you should not move patients unless it is necessary to perform _____ or remove them from a dangerous situation.

10. The three basic types of splints are rigid, soft, and _____.

Short Answer

Complete this section with short written answers using the space provided.

1. Name the four primary functions of the skeletal system.

_____

_____

2. Name the three major types of injuries to the musculoskeletal system.

_____

_____

3. Name four signs of injury you should look for during a visual examination of the limb.

_____

_____

4. What two questions should you ask a patient who has a limb injury?

_____

_____

5. Name two ways to check for adequate circulation in an injured limb.

_____

_____

6. Name three key signs and symptoms of a spinal injury.

_____

_____

7. Name four things you should always check on an injured limb both before and after splinting.

_____

_____

8. What are the five steps for splinting a forearm injury with a SAM splint?

_____

_____

9. Describe the three types of mechanism of injury and give an example of each type.

_____

_____

10. List the seven areas of the skeletal system.

_____

_____

11. Describe how you would splint an injury to the elbow.

_____

_____

12. Describe four signs or symptoms of a head injury.

_____

_____

13. Describe the treatment for a head injury.

_____

_____

14. List three signs or symptoms of extremity injuries.

_____

_____

You Make the Call

The following scenarios provide an opportunity to explore the concerns associated with patient management. Read the scenarios and answer the questions to the best of your ability.

1. You are dispatched to the scene of a "long fall." When you arrive, you find a 26-year-old man lying on the snow next to a ladder leaning against the house and Christmas lights hanging from the front of the house. His right leg is deformed. What should you do?

_____

_____

_____

2. Your unit is dispatched to an altercation at a local bar. When you arrive, you see one man sitting outside the bar with a towel on his head. You notice the towel is covered with blood; the patient tells you he was struck in the head with a beer bottle. The bartender tells you that two men were fighting in the bar and that one of the men left the scene before your arrival. What should you do?

_____

_____

_____

Skills

Skill Drills

Test your knowledge of this skill by filling in the correct words in the photo caption.

Skill Drill 14-1: Checking Circulation, Sensation, and Movement in an Injured Extremity

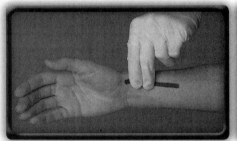 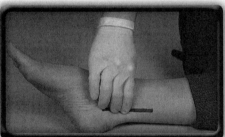 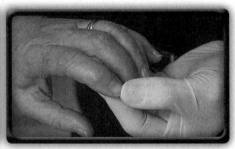

1. Check for circulation. If upper extremity injury, check _____ pulse.

2. If lower extremity injury, check _____ _____ pulse.

3. Test _____ _____ on finger/toe of injured limb.

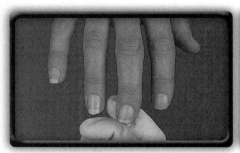 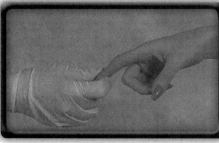 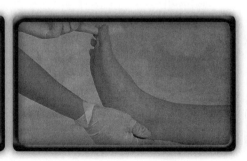

4. Release pressure. _____ color should return.

5. Check for _____ at fingertips.

6. Check for _____ at toes.

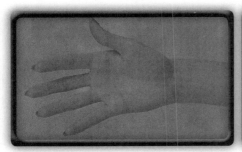
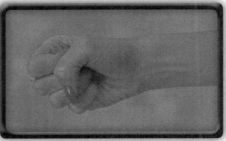

7. Check for _____ of the upper extremities by asking the patient to open and close the fist.

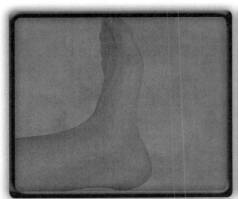
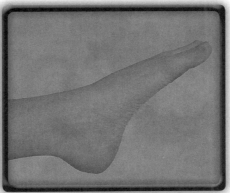

8. Check for _____ of the lower extremities by asking the patient to extend and flex the ankle.

Skill Drill 14-4: Applying a Traction Splint

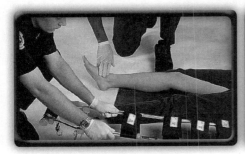
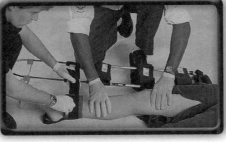
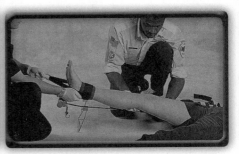

1. Place the splint beside the _____ limb, adjust the splint to the proper length, and prepare the straps.

2. Support the injured limb as your partner fastens the _____ _____ about the foot and ankle.

3. Continue to support the limb as your partner applies gentle _____ to the _____ _____ and foot.

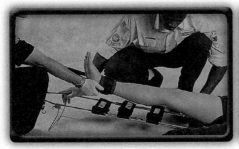

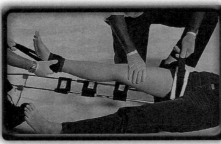

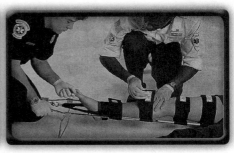

4. Slide the _____ into position under the injured limb.

5. Pad the _____ and fasten the strap around the _____.

6. Connect the loops of the ankle hitch to the end of the splint as your partner continues to maintain _____. Fasten the support straps so that the _____ is securely held in the splint.

Skill Drill 14-8: Removing the Mask on a Sports Helmet

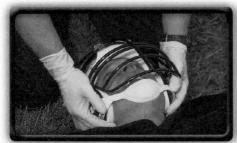

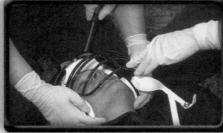

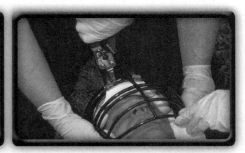

1. Stabilize the patient's head and helmet in a(n) _____, in-line position. Then remove the mask in one of the following two ways.

2. Use a(n) _____ to unscrew the retaining clips for the face mask or perform Step 3.

3. Use a(n) _____ _____ designed for cutting retaining clips.

Skill Drill 14-9: Removing a Helmet

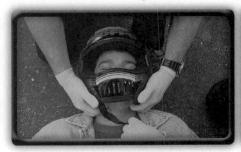

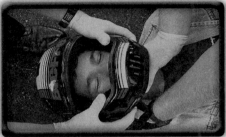

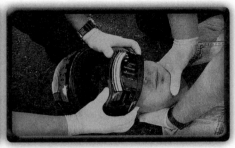

1. Kneel down at the patient's head and open the face shield to assess the _____ and _____. Stabilize the helmet by placing your hands on either side of it, ensuring that your fingers are on the patient's _____ _____ to prevent movement of the head. Your partner can then loosen the strap.

2. Your partner should place one hand on the patient's _____ _____ and the other behind the _____ at the occiput.

3. Gently slip the helmet off about _____ and then stop.

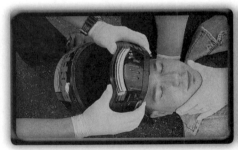

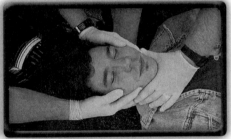

4. Your partner slides his or her hand from the occiput to the _____ of the head to prevent the head from snapping back once the helmet is removed.

5. With your partner's hand in place, remove the helmet and stabilize the _____ _____. Apply a cervical collar and then secure the patient to a long backboard.

General Knowledge

Matching

Match each of the items in the left column to the appropriate definition in the right column.

_____	**1.** Placenta	**A.** Muscular organ that holds and nourishes the developing fetus
_____	**2.** Miscarriage	**B.** Bloody mucus plug that is discharged from the vagina when labor begins
_____	**3.** Contractions	**C.** Rubber or plastic device used for gentle suction with newborns and infants
_____	**4.** Bloody show	**D.** Delivery in which the infant's buttocks appear first rather than the head
_____	**5.** Fetus	**E.** Life-support system of the fetus (commonly called the afterbirth)
_____	**6.** Uterus	**F.** Amniotic fluid–filled sac
_____	**7.** Bulb syringe	**G.** Delivery of the fetus before it is mature enough to survive outside the womb
_____	**8.** Bag of waters	**H.** Muscular movements of the uterus
_____	**9.** Crowning	**I.** Developing infant in the uterus
_____	**10.** Breech presentation	**J.** Appearance of the infant's head through the birth canal

Multiple Choice

Read each item carefully and then select the one best response.

_____ **1.** If the infant's head is crowning, that means the infant will be born:

    A. breech.

    B. in a matter of minutes.

    C. with breathing difficulties.

    D. with a prolapsed cord.

_____ **2.** When you assess for crowning, you notice the umbilical cord protruding through the vagina. Your care should include all of the following EXCEPT:

    A. arranging for immediate transport.

    B. laying the mother on her right side.

    C. raising the mother's hips.

    D. administering oxygen to the mother.

_____ **3.** The first thing you must decide during a childbirth situation is whether you:

    A. are calm enough to handle the situation.

    B. have the proper equipment to deal with the situation.

    C. have time to transport the mother to the hospital before delivery.

    D. can rely on the mother to know enough about childbirth to help you with the delivery.

_____ **4.** A young mother in labor tells you that this is her first pregnancy, that she has been having contractions for the past 8 hours, and that her water broke some time ago. You should prepare to:

    A. deliver the infant because birth is imminent after 8 hours of labor.

    B. ask about discharge of bloody mucus because delivery will be a long time off unless this has also occurred.

    C. transport her immediately to the nearest hospital because the length of her labor indicates a serious problem with the pregnancy.

    D. time the contractions and check to see if the head is crowning before transporting her to a hospital.

_____ **5.** The mother's contractions are 4 minutes apart, and the infant's head is not crowning yet. In what stage of labor is the mother?

    A. First

    B. Second

    C. Third

    D. Between the second and the third

_____ **6.** A woman in labor is 30 minutes from the nearest hospital, and an ambulance has not yet been called when you arrive on the scene. You should:

    A. transport the mother immediately in your own vehicle.

    B. prepare for the delivery, given the mother's condition.

    C. call an ambulance but prepare for the delivery.

    D. call an ambulance but transport the mother in your own vehicle if contractions start occurring closer together.

_____ **7.** The best way to detect crowning is to:

    A. observe the vaginal opening during a contraction.

    B. ask the mother if she feels the infant's head at her vaginal opening.

    C. wait until a contraction has ended and then observe the vaginal opening.

    D. use your gloved fingertips to feel gently for the infant's head at the vaginal opening.

_____ **8.** To prevent the infant's head from emerging too rapidly, you should tell the mother to:

    A. stop pushing.

    B. hold her breath.

    C. push more slowly.

    D. relax her abdominal muscles.

_____ **9.** A mother in the second stage of labor says she has to move her bowels. You should:

    A. help her to the bathroom.

    B. find a container she can use as a bedpan.

    C. ask her if she is sure it is not just the pressure of the infant that she is feeling.

    D. tell her she is only feeling the pressure of the infant and should not try to relieve the feeling now.

_____ **10.** You should handle the umbilical cord when:

    A. it is caught in the vagina.

    B. it is wrapped around the infant's neck.

    C. delivery of the placenta is delayed.

    D. you pull on it to deliver the placenta.

_____ **11.** After an infant has been delivered, you should immediately:

    A. try to get the infant to cry.

    B. invert the infant.

    C. begin mouth-to-mouth resuscitation.

    D. clear the infant's nose and mouth.

_____ **12.** If a newborn shows no signs of life and has an unpleasant odor, you should first:

    A. begin resuscitation efforts.

    B. try to keep the newborn warm.

    C. tell the mother she has had a miscarriage.

    D. provide physical care and psychological support for the mother.

_____ **13.** A mother tells you that she was pregnant for only 7 months with the infant you have just helped deliver. You should recognize that the infant will likely:

    A. require CPR.

    B. have bluish skin.

    C. need to be kept especially warm.

    D. have a larger head than a full-term infant.

_____ **14.** The muscular organ that holds and nourishes a developing fetus is called the:

    A. placenta.

    B. vagina.

    C. uterus.

    D. fallopian tube.

_____ **15.** The process of delivering an infant is called:

    A. crowning.

    B. labor.

    C. contractions.

    D. fetus.

_____ **16.** During the first stage of labor:

    A. the bloody show occurs.

    B. the crowning of the infant's head occurs.

    C. the pregnant woman should not be transported.

    D. all of the above.

_____ **17.** You usually have time to transport a woman in labor when the contractions are more than how many minutes apart?

    A. 4 minutes

    B. 5 minutes

    C. 6 minutes

    D. 7 minutes

_____ **18.** The infant's head is beginning to emerge. Which of the following should occur?

    A. The woman should stop pushing.

    B. The woman should push harder.

    C. The woman should breathe rapidly.

    D. Both A and C.

_____ **19.** After the placenta is delivered:

    A. place it in a bag and discard it with the medical waste.

    B. place it in a plastic bag and transport it to the hospital for examination.

    C. place it in a bag of sterile water.

    D. keep it at a lower level than the infant.

_____ **20.** Which of the following statements regarding a breech birth is false?

    A. You should arrange for immediate transport to an appropriate medical facility.

    B. A breech birth slows the labor.

    C. There will be crowning of the infant's head.

    D. A breech birth can result in injury to the newborn and the mother.

_____ **21.** If an infant does not begin breathing independently after delivery, the EMR may:

    A. suction the mouth and nose.

    B. tilt the infant's head down and to the side.

    C. gently stimulate the soles of the feet and/or back.

    D. all of the above.

_____ **22.** When timing contractions, you should:

    A. time the interval between contractions.

    B. time the contraction cycles from the beginning of one contraction to the beginning of the next.

    C. time the contraction cycles from the end of one contraction to the end of the next.

    D. time the contraction cycles from the beginning of one contraction to the end of the next.

_____ **23.** You should begin chest compressions on a newborn if the pulse rate is less than:
  A. 100 beats per minute.
  B. 80 beats per minute.
  C. 70 beats per minute.
  D. 60 beats per minute.

_____ **24.** Vaginal bleeding in a pregnant woman is often the first sign of:
  A. labor.
  B. stillborn delivery.
  C. miscarriage.
  D. ectopic pregnancy.

_____ **25.** If the newborn is surrounded by the bag of waters:
  A. carefully break the bag and push it away from the nose and mouth of the newborn.
  B. leave the bag in place and wait for ALS assistance.
  C. leave the bag in place and transport immediately to an appropriate medical facility.
  D. carefully puncture the bag to remove the fluid, but leave the bag in place.

_____ **26.** Which of the following is false when preparing for a delivery?
  A. You should elevate the mother's hip 2" to 4" with pillows and blankets.
  B. You must maintain a sterile environment when preparing for delivery.
  C. You should have plenty of clean towels ready to cover the infant.
  D. If you do not have a sterile delivery kit, use the gloves from your EMR life support kit.

_____ **27.** If the mother is bleeding severely:
  A. place one or more clean sanitary pads at the opening of the vagina.
  B. elevate the legs and hips.
  C. arrange for rapid transport to the hospital by ambulance.
  D. all of the above.

True/False

If you believe the statement to be more true than false, write the letter "T" in the space provided. If you believe the statement to be more false than true, write the letter "F."

_____ **1.** Assisting in childbirth means no more than receiving the infant as it is delivered and making sure it begins to breathe.

_____ **2.** Wearing kitchen gloves for a delivery is better than wearing no gloves at all.

_____ **3.** You must pull the infant's body out of the mother after the head has emerged.

_____ **4.** If an infant turns to the side after the head emerges, you should try to correct its position.

_____ **5.** If instead of normal crowning, you see a breech presentation, you should prepare for immediate delivery.

_____ **6.** In the case of a breech birth, it may be necessary to gently pull the infant to assist with delivery.

_____ **7.** Prolapse of the umbilical cord means that the cord comes out of the vagina before the infant is born and needs to be pushed back into the vagina until delivery.

_____ **8.** If it looks like a woman has lost about 2 cups of blood during delivery, you should rapidly transport her to the hospital.

_____ **9.** If a miscarriage occurs, all of the tissues that have been passed from the vagina should be saved.

_____ **10.** A stillborn fetus is one who does not begin breathing independently within 1 minute of delivery.

_____ **11.** Normal labor consists of five distinct stages.

_____ **12.** A pregnant woman in either of the first two stages of labor should be transported.

_____ **13.** In the second stage of labor, you will see the infant's head crowning during contractions.

_____ **14.** Stage three of labor involves delivery of the placenta.

_____ **15.** Contractions during labor are timed by calculating the amount of time between the end of one contraction and the beginning of the next.

_____ **16.** A woman who has previously given birth will have more time to reach the hospital than a woman who is pregnant with her first child.

_____ **17.** Transport of a pregnant woman in labor should not be attempted if the contractions are less than 3 minutes apart or if the infant's head is crowning.

_____ **18.** Newspapers, towels, aluminum foil, and shower curtains can be used as equipment during a home delivery.

_____ **19.** Face and eye protection are not necessary during delivery.

_____ **20.** Delivery of an infant should not be attempted unless a prepackaged delivery kit is available.

_____ **21.** To avoid contamination during delivery, a woman who is in labor should be encouraged to use the bathroom for bowel movements.

_____ **22.** It is important that the umbilical cord is cut as soon as the infant is breathing independently.

_____ **23.** Massaging the uterus will help it become firm and will help stop bleeding.

_____ **24.** If an infant does not breathe on its own within 1 minute after birth, CPR should begin immediately.

_____ **25.** When an infant is born in an unbroken bag of waters, you should carefully break the bag, push it away from the infant's nose and mouth, and suction the infant's nose and mouth.

_____ **26.** If a pregnant woman is involved in a motor vehicle collision, she should be transported to the hospital on her left side rather than on her back.

_____ **27.** During normal childbirth, the mother loses about 3 to 4 cups of blood.

_____ **28.** Nursing the newborn after delivery is associated with an increase in hemorrhaging.

Labeling

Label the following diagrams with the correct terms.

1. Anatomy of a Pregnant Woman

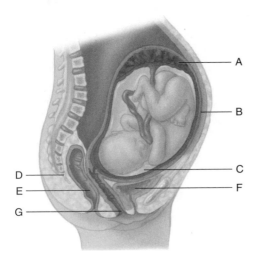

A. _____

B. _____

C. _____

D. _____

E. _____

F. _____

G. _____

2. Phases of the Second Stage of Labor

A. _____

B. _____

C. _____

D. _____

A

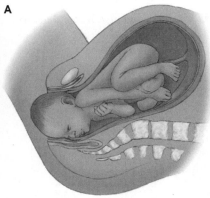

B

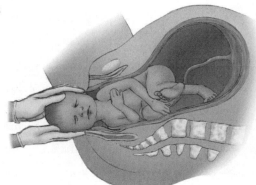

C

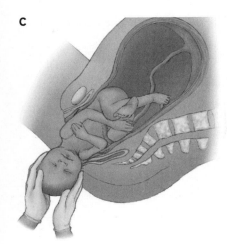

D

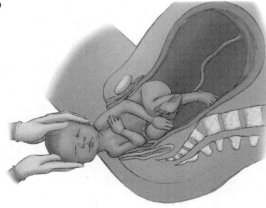

Crossword Puzzle

Use the clues in the column to complete the crossword puzzle.

Across

4. The distal or terminal ending of the gastrointestinal tract.
5. Infants delivered before 36 weeks of gestation or who weigh less than 5 pounds at birth.
8. The process of delivering an infant.
9. The vagina and the lower part of the uterus.
10. A pregnancy that occurs outside the uterus, usually in a fallopian tube; usually terminates with the rupture of the fallopian tube.

Down

1. The opening through which the infant emerges.
2. Aspirating (sucking out) fluid by mechanical means.
3. Muscular organ that holds and nourishes the developing fetus; also called the uterus.
6. Ropelike attachment between the pregnant woman and fetus; nourishment and waste products pass to and from the fetus and the woman through this cord.
7. A(n) _____ umbilical cord appears before the infant does; the infant's head may compress the cord and cut off all circulation.

Critical Thinking

Fill-in-the-Blank

Read each item carefully and then complete the statement by filling in the missing words.

1. The _____, or afterbirth, draws nutrients from the wall of the mother's uterus.

2. Stage _____ of labor is when the mother's body prepares for birth.

3. To determine when the infant's head is _____, you must observe the vaginal opening during a contraction.

4. Your primary purpose is to _____ in the delivery of the infant.

5. In a normal delivery, there is no need to cut the _____ cord.

6. In a(n) _____ birth, the infant's buttocks come down the birth canal first, rather than the head.

7. A(n) _____, also called a spontaneous abortion, is the delivery of an incomplete or underdeveloped fetus.

8. In the event of _____ births, another set of labor contractions will begin shortly after the delivery of the first infant.

9. Contractions should be timed from the _____ of one contraction to the beginning of the next contraction.

10. Any infant weighing less than 5 pounds or delivered before 36 weeks of pregnancy is considered _____.

Short Answer

Complete this section with short written answers using the space provided.

1. Describe the three stages of labor.

_____

_____

2. List the seven questions you should ask yourself when deciding if there is enough time to reach the hospital before delivery.

_____

_____

3. What is the appropriate procedure for putting on sterile gloves?

_____

_____

4. Name three important steps of care after a miscarriage.

_____

_____

You Make the Call

The following scenarios provide an opportunity to explore the concerns associated with patient management. Read the scenarios and answer the questions to the best of your ability.

1. You arrive on the scene and find a 32-year-old woman who tells you she is $8\frac{1}{2}$ months pregnant. This is her fifth pregnancy, and she's afraid she won't be able to make it to the hospital in time. She tells you her last labor lasted less than 2 hours. She is having frequent contractions. What should you do?

_____

_____

_____

2. You arrive at the scene of a 27-year-old woman complaining of severe abdominal pain. The patient denies being pregnant, although she reports that she missed her last menstrual period. The patient is pale with a rapid pulse and decreased blood pressure. What is most likely wrong with this patient, and what is the proper treatment?

_____

_____

_____

Skills

Skill Drills

Test your knowledge of this skill by filling in the correct words in the photo caption.

Skill Drill 15-2: Resuscitating a Newborn

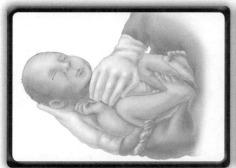

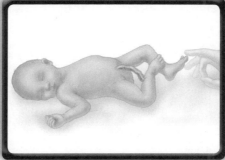

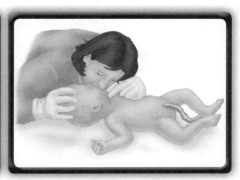

1. Tilt the infant so the _____ is down and to the side to clear the airway.

2. Gently snap or flick your fingers on the _____ of the infant's feet.

3. Begin _____ _____.

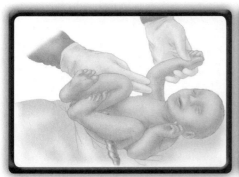

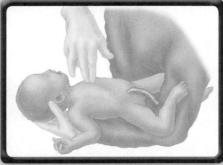

4. Check for a(n) _____ pulse.

5. Begin _____ _____ using the middle and ring fingers.

Pediatric Emergencies

General Knowledge

Matching

Match each of the items in the left column to the appropriate definition in the right column.

_____ **1.** Drowning

_____ **2.** Mottling

_____ **3.** Suctioning

_____ **4.** Epilepsy

_____ **5.** Asthma

_____ **6.** Croup

_____ **7.** Epiglottitis

A. Severe inflammation and swelling of the epiglottis

B. Patchy skin discoloration caused by too little or too much circulation

C. Submersion in water that results in suffocation or respiratory impairment

D. Acute spasm of the smaller air passages marked by labored breathing and wheezing

E. Disease manifested by seizures; caused by abnormal focus of electrical activity in the brain

F. Aspirating fluid by mechanical means

G. Causes a barking cough, hoarseness, and a harsh, high-pitched breathing sound

Multiple Choice

Read each item carefully and then select the one best response.

_____ **1.** Although the technique used to open the airway of an infant is the same as that used for an adult, you should make sure that the infant's head is placed in what position?

A. Neutral

B. Extended

C. Hyperextended

D. Turned to the right side

_____ **2.** To remove a foreign object from an infant's airway, you should alternate chest thrusts with:

A. CPR.

B. back slaps.

C. rescue breathing.

D. the Heimlich maneuver.

_____ **3.** Rapid, shallow breathing and/or a rapid, weak pulse should immediately signal that a child is in:

A. shock.

B. a coma.

C. cardiac arrest.

D. the middle of a convulsion.

_____ **4.** You are called to the scene of a motor vehicle crash in which a man and a woman are killed, but their 6-month-old son is alive in a car seat in the back seat. You decide to remove the baby from the car because you smell gasoline. You should try to remove the baby:

A. after EMS personnel arrive.

B. while he is still in the car seat.

C. only after you take him out of the car seat.

D. only if you can place him on an infant backboard.

_____ **5.** Which of the following is not an indication of child abuse?

    A. Withdrawn, fearful, or even hostile child

    B. History of "accidents"

    C. Spider bite

    D. Bruises in various stages of healing

_____ **6.** Which of the following is considered a key pediatric medical emergency or illness?

    A. Drowning

    B. Road rash

    C. Headache

    D. Coughing

_____ **7.** A hoarse, whooping noise during inhalation and a seal-like barking cough are symptoms of which respiratory illness?

    A. Asthma

    B. Croup

    C. Pneumonia

    D. Allergies

_____ **8.** What are the four essential skills required for treating respiratory emergencies in infants and children?

    A. CPR, maintaining normal body temperature, use of oxygen, and rescue breathing

    B. CPR, use of a defibrillator, splinting of extremities, and starting an IV

    C. Opening the airway, basic life support, suctioning, and use of airway adjuncts

    D. Use of oxygen, application of a backboard, assessing breath sounds, and chest compressions

_____ **9.** Which of the following is not a characteristic used for evaluating work of breathing?

    A. Abnormal breath sounds

    B. Facial color

    C. Abnormal positioning

    D. Flaring

_____ **10.** When caring for seriously ill or injured pediatric patients, it is important to check the vital signs every _____ minutes.

    A. 2

    B. 5

    C. 10

    D. 20

_____ **11.** Children lose relatively more heat than adults do because:

    A. they tend to wear fewer outer garments.

    B. they use more energy.

    C. they have a greater surface area relative to the mass of their body.

    D. all of the above.

_____ **12.** When performing patient assessment on a child, you should pay special attention to:

    A. work of breathing.

    B. circulation to the skin.

    C. appearance.

    D. all of the above.

_____ **13.** High body temperatures in children are often accompanied by:

    A. wheezing and dry skin.

    B. unresponsiveness and a lackluster appearance.

    C. flushed, red skin; sweating; and restlessness.

    D. decreased pulse rate.

_____ **14.** The normal respiratory rate for a newborn is _____ breaths per minute.
   A. 30 to 60
   B. 20 to 30
   C. 18 to 22
   D. 12 to 18

_____ **15.** The normal pulse rate for a newborn is _____ beats per minute.
   A. 90 to 180
   B. 140
   C. 120
   D. 100 to 160

_____ **16.** The normal respiratory rate for a 10-year-old is _____ breaths per minute.
   A. 30 to 60
   B. 25 to 50
   C. 15 to 20
   D. 12 to 16

_____ **17.** The most common cause of circulatory failure in a child is:
   A. traumatic injury.
   B. sudden infant death syndrome.
   C. respiratory failure.
   D. drowning.

_____ **18.** To select the proper size of oral airway for a child or an infant, you should measure:
   A. from the earlobe to the jaw.
   B. from the earlobe to the nose.
   C. from the jaw to the corner of the mouth.
   D. from the earlobe to the corner of the mouth.

_____ **19.** For a severe airway obstruction in a conscious child:
   A. begin with blind finger sweeps.
   B. use the Heimlich maneuver.
   C. use the chest-thrust maneuver.
   D. hyperextend the neck and recheck for breathing.

_____ **20.** For an airway obstruction in an unconscious infant:
   A. activate the EMS system.
   B. use finger sweeps only if you see a foreign object.
   C. open the airway with the head tilt–chin lift maneuver.
   D. all of the above.

_____ **21.** Which of the following is not a sign of respiratory distress in a child?
   A. A breathing rate of more than 30 to 40 breaths per minute in infants
   B. Retraction of the skin between the ribs and around the neck muscles
   C. Altered mental status
   D. Nasal flaring on each breath

_____ **22.** A sign of respiratory failure in a child is:
   A. a respiratory rate of more than 30 breaths per minute.
   B. combativeness or restlessness.
   C. stridor, a high-pitched sound on inspiration.
   D. limp muscle tone.

_____ **23.** Altered mental status in children can be caused by:
  A. head trauma.
  B. infection.
  C. low blood glucose level.
  D. all of the above.

_____ **24.** The main signs and symptoms of croup include all of the following EXCEPT:
  A. noisy, whooping inhalations.
  B. a seal-like barking cough.
  C. fright or anxiety.
  D. history of a recent or current cold.

_____ **25.** Epiglottitis usually occurs in children from _____ of age.
  A. 3 to 6 months
  B. 3 to 6 years
  C. 1 to 3 months
  D. 1 to 3 years

_____ **26.** The signs and symptoms of epiglottitis include all of the following EXCEPT:
  A. the child is drooling.
  B. the child cannot swallow.
  C. the child is lying down.
  D. the child is anxious and frightened.

_____ **27.** If you encounter a child with a fever above 104°F (40°C), you should:
  A. fan the child to cool him or her down.
  B. attempt to reduce the high temperature by undressing the child.
  C. protect the child during any seizure that might result.
  D. all of the above.

_____ **28.** Appropriate care for a child while he or she is having a seizure includes which of the following?
  A. Inserting an oral airway to keep the airway open
  B. Placing the child on the floor or bed to prevent injury
  C. Raising the child's legs to increase blood flow to the brain
  D. All of the above

_____ **29.** Appendicitis is most often seen in people between the ages of:
  A. 10 and 25 years.
  B. 5 and 10 years.
  C. 20 and 35 years.
  D. 35 and 50 years.

_____ **30.** Poisoning by absorption occurs when a poisonous substance enters the body through:
  A. the mouth.
  B. injection.
  C. the skin.
  D. the eyes.

_____ **31.** Poisoning by ingestion occurs when a poisonous substance enters the body through:
  A. the mouth.
  B. the skin.
  C. injection.
  D. the eyes.

_____ **32.** Typical injuries you should look for when a child has been hit by a motor vehicle include:
   A. injuries to the legs.
   B. injuries to the chest.
   C. injuries to the head.
   D. all of the above.

_____ **33.** Signs and symptoms of traumatic shock include all of the following EXCEPT:
   A. increased blood pressure.
   B. cool, clammy skin.
   C. rapid, weak pulse.
   D. rapid or shallow respirations.

_____ **34.** Which of the following statements regarding parents is false?
   A. Many parents can become emotionally distraught by large amounts of blood.
   B. A child's parents or caregivers can be either allies or a potential problem.
   C. Parents are generally unable to tell you how the child's behavior is different.
   D. Children get many of their behavioral cues from their parents.

_____ **35.** All of the following illustrate differences between the adult and pediatric airway EXCEPT:
   A. a child's tongue is relatively larger than the tongue of an adult.
   B. an adult's airway is more flexible than a child's airway.
   C. a child's airway is smaller in relation to the rest of the body.
   D. infants breathe only through their noses for at least the first 6 months of their lives.

True/False

If you believe the statement to be more true than false, write the letter "T" in the space provided. If you believe the statement to be more false than true, write the letter "F."

_____ **1.** Managing a pediatric emergency can be one of the most stressful situations you face as an EMR.

_____ **2.** Calming a parent is sometimes the best way to calm a child.

_____ **3.** You should avoid telling a child when some parts of the treatment will be painful because the child will only become more nervous.

_____ **4.** When a child is poisoned, you should try to identify the poison and how much the child has swallowed to report to the doctor or the poison control center.

_____ **5.** You should always try to induce vomiting in a child who has swallowed poison.

_____ **6.** A child who has swallowed poison may require rescue breathing or even CPR.

_____ **7.** A high fever always means a child is seriously ill.

_____ **8.** A child who has signs of dehydration needs to be examined by a physician.

_____ **9.** A child with a high fever who is covered with blankets may actually go into convulsions.

_____ **10.** Even if you are able to reduce a high fever, the child must be seen by a physician.

_____ **11.** Trauma is the number one killer of children.

_____ **12.** A child shows signs of shock much sooner than an adult.

_____ **13.** You should always look for head and abdominal injuries in a child who has been struck by a motor vehicle.

_____ **14.** You may skip a full-body assessment of a seriously injured child who is too young to understand or respond to your questions about his or her injuries.

_____ **15.** The only time you should attempt to remove an object that is partially blocking a child's airway is when you can see the object in the child's mouth and can remove it easily.

_____ **16.** If you are not sure whether you should remove an object partially blocking a child's airway or if you cannot see the object, you should transport the child to an appropriate medical facility as soon as possible without trying to remove the object.

_____ **17.** Talking and explaining what you are doing to a child who has a partially blocked airway is likely to make the child more anxious.

_____ **18.** Risks at home that can increase the risk of drowning for young children include buckets of water, toilet bowls, washbowls, and bathtubs.

_____ **19.** Children's pulse rates become faster with each degree of body temperature increase.

_____ **20.** Three-year-olds have faster pulse rates than newborns.

_____ **21.** The head tilt–chin lift technique can be used for children who have sustained an injury to the neck or head.

_____ **22.** Use a bulb syringe to suction the nose of a child.

_____ **23.** Never transport a child in the arms of a parent because parents are too emotional and may excite the child.

_____ **24.** Performing mouth-to-mask ventilations is an appropriate intervention for a child experiencing respiratory failure.

_____ **25.** Respiratory distress in a child often leads quickly to respiratory failure.

_____ **26.** It is important to determine the cause of a child's altered mental status before treating the symptoms.

_____ **27.** When experiencing an asthma attack, a child can exhale easily but has difficulty inhaling.

_____ **28.** When experiencing an asthma attack, a child should be placed in a sitting position.

_____ **29.** Croup is an infection of the upper airway that usually occurs in infants from 4 to 6 months of age.

_____ **30.** Epiglottitis is the most severe of the three major childhood respiratory problems.

_____ **31.** Epiglottitis usually occurs in children from 1 to 3 years of age.

_____ **32.** Although childhood seizures can be frightening, they are not usually dangerous.

_____ **33.** Prolonged vomiting can produce severe dehydration in a child.

_____ **34.** A patient with appendicitis usually experiences pain originating in the belly button area of the stomach.

_____ **35.** SIDS is usually the result of chronic child abuse.

_____ **36.** The three components of the Pediatric Assessment Triangle are appearance, work of breathing, and circulation to skin.

_____ **37.** By looking at the types of trauma a child has experienced, you can better anticipate the types of injuries a child may have sustained.

_____ **38.** In dealing with the parents of an abused child, you should conduct yourself in a judgmental manner to get them to confess.

Crossword Puzzle

Use the clues in the column to complete the crossword puzzle.

Across

2. CPR for infants (younger than 1 year) involves giving gentle rescue breaths, using mouth-to-_____ ventilations.

4. These sessions are organized after especially emotional incidents involving children to allow EMRs to express their feelings, learn coping strategies, and maintain a healthy approach to future calls.

7. Good eye contact, good muscle tone, and good color are an assessment of this part of the Pediatric Assessment Triangle.

8. The normal respiratory rate for a patient in this age group is 12 to 20 breaths per minute.

10. The _____ maneuver is a series of manual thrusts to the chest to relieve upper airway obstruction; used in the treatment of infants, pregnant women, or extremely obese people.

Down

1. Bluish discoloration of the skin and mucous membranes.

3. Signs and symptoms of respiratory _____ include a respiratory rate of more than 60 breaths per minute in infants and more than 30 to 40 breaths per minute in children.

5. Signs and symptoms of respiratory _____ include a respiratory rate of fewer than 20 breaths per minute in infants and fewer than 10 breaths per minute in children.

6. When positioning the patient's airway for insertion of an oral airway, if the pediatric patient has a traumatic injury, the _____ maneuver should be used.

9. An assessment tool that measures the severity of a child's illness or injury by evaluating the child's appearance, work of breathing, and circulation to the skin.

Critical Thinking

Fill-in-the-Blank

Read each item carefully and then complete the statement by filling in the missing words.

1. SIDS usually occurs in infants between the ages of _____ and _____.

2. _____ is a characteristic of circulation to the skin that demonstrates white or pale skin or mucous membranes.

3. The _____ _____ _____ is an easy-to-remember tool that allows you to quickly form a general impression of a child and incorporates an assessment of appearance, work of breathing, and circulation to the skin.

4. Normal vital signs for a newborn are a pulse rate of _____ beats per minute and a respiratory rate of _____ breaths per minute.

5. The number one killer of children is _____.

6. You can usually relieve a(n) _____ airway obstruction by placing the child on his or her _____, tilting the head, and lifting the _____ in the usual manner.

7. Asthma can occur in children older than _____.

8. _____ is the second most common cause of accidental death among children 5 years of age or younger in the United States.

9. The most dangerous heat-related illness in children is _____.

10. Prolonged vomiting and diarrhea may produce severe _____.

Short Answer
Complete this section with short written answers using the space provided.

1. Name the three vital signs you should closely watch when conducting a primary assessment of an infant or a young child.

_____

_____

2. Name three objects a child might swallow that would have to be removed at the hospital.

_____

_____

3. Name the three most important things you can do for a child who has traumatic injuries.

_____

_____

4. Describe how you would care for a child who has heatstroke.

_____

_____

5. Name four steps in caring for a child who has a high fever.

_____

_____

6. What is the most important rule of thumb when responding to cases of abdominal pain in children?

_____

_____

7. List four signs and symptoms of possible neglect in a child.

_____

_____

8. What should you do if you suspect that a child has been sexually or physically abused, but the parents refuse to allow you to arrange to have the child seen by a physician?

_____

_____

9. Under what circumstances should you begin CPR on an infant who has been found dead for no apparent reason?

_____

_____

You Make the Call

The following scenarios provide an opportunity to explore the concerns associated with patient management. Read the scenarios and answer the questions to the best of your ability.

1. As you are returning to your station, you notice a small child dart from the curb, right into the path of an oncoming car. The child is struck by the vehicle. He is approximately 2 years old, and the car was moving at a speed of approximately 30 miles per hour. What should you do?

_____

_____

_____

2. You respond to a local residence for an unresponsive child. When you arrive on scene, you find a child lying next to a swimming pool, being attended to by her parents. The mother is hysterical and is screaming for you to save her child. The child is unresponsive and does not appear to be breathing. What should you do?

_____

_____

_____

Skills

Skill Drills

Test your knowledge of this skill by filling in the correct words in the photo caption.

Skill Drill 16-1: Inserting an Oral Airway in a Child

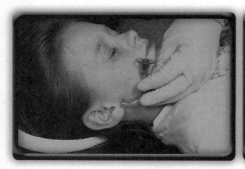
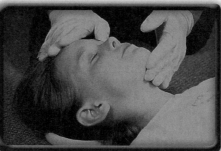
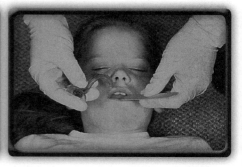

1. Select the proper size oral airway by measuring from the patient's _____ to the corner of the _____.

2. _____ the pediatric patient's airway with the appropriate method.

3. Depress the patient's tongue and press the tongue _____ and away from the _____ of the mouth. Follow the anatomic curve of the roof of the patient's mouth to _____ the airway into place.

Geriatric Emergencies

General Knowledge

Matching

Match each of the items in the left column to the appropriate definition in the right column.

_____ **1.** Alzheimer disease

_____ **2.** Osteoporosis

_____ **3.** Suicide

_____ **4.** Hospice

_____ **5.** Senile dementia

_____ **6.** Depression

_____ **7.** Dementia

A. Intentionally causing one's own death

B. Chronic progressive dementia that accounts for 60% of all dementia

C. An interdisciplinary program designed to reduce or eliminate pain and address the physical, spiritual, social, and economic needs of terminally ill patients

D. Abnormal brittleness of the bones caused by loss of calcium; affected bones fracture easily

E. Progressive irreversible decline in mental functioning

F. General term for dementia that occurs in older people

G. Persistent feelings of sadness, hopelessness, and decreased interest in daily activities

Multiple Choice

Read each item carefully and then select the one best response.

_____ **1.** An elderly man seems hesitant and unsure of himself when you ask him to walk from his bed to a nearby chair. You should:

    A. offer him your arm for support.

    B. prepare to move him yourself because he is probably senile.

    C. pull him gently in the direction you want him to go because he is probably hard of hearing.

    D. ask him again more slowly because, like other older people, he thinks more slowly.

_____ **2.** Fractures are more common among the elderly because of a condition called:

    A. diabetes.

    B. senility.

    C. arthritis.

    D. osteoporosis.

_____ **3.** As you begin to examine an elderly woman who is dressed in several layers of clothing, you should:

    A. take her vital signs only.

    B. remove all of her clothing to allow for a thorough examination.

    C. remove as much of the clothing as you need to examine her properly.

    D. perform a less-than-complete physical examination.

_____ **4.** A man who points at his ear and shakes his head "no" may be trying to tell you that:

    A. he is deaf.

    B. he is senile.

    C. he wants you to repeat what you said.

    D. you should not speak to him.

_____   **5.** The most important factor to consider when caring for a blind patient is that you will:

    A. have to watch the person's guide dog.

    B. have trouble reading the person's facial expressions.

    C. need to allow the patient to touch you more than a sighted patient would.

    D. need to explain more to the patient about what you are doing and what is happening.

_____   **6.** A geriatric patient is commonly defined as a patient who is more than _____ years of age.

    A. 50

    B. 55

    C. 60

    D. 65

_____   **7.** Concerns particular to geriatric patients include:

    A. sensory changes, such as hearing loss and vision impairment.

    B. changes in mobility.

    C. changes in medical conditions.

    D. all of the above.

_____   **8.** Which of the following does not affect the natural aging process?

    A. Heredity

    B. Environment

    C. Stress level

    D. Diet

_____   **9.** If an older patient loses his eyeglasses during an emergency and is anxious, you should:

    A. search and try to find them.

    B. explain what is going on for the patient who can no longer see.

    C. calm the patient and tell him not to worry about it.

    D. ask if the patient has the original prescription and try to obtain new eyeglasses.

_____   **10.** A common site for fractures in geriatric patients is the:

    A. neck.

    B. ankle.

    C. wrist.

    D. knee.

_____   **11.** Cardiovascular changes in geriatric patients place them at risk for cardiac diseases such as all of the following EXCEPT:

    A. congestive heart failure.

    B. chronic obstructive pulmonary disease.

    C. angina.

    D. heart attack.

_____   **12.** Which of the following is not a common cause of altered mental status in a geriatric patient?

    A. Dementia

    B. Lack of adequate oxygen to the brain

    C. Low blood glucose level

    D. Hypothermia

True/False

If you believe the statement to be more true than false, write the letter "T" in the space provided. If you believe the statement to be more false than true, write the letter "F."

_____ **1.** Cancer is a frequent cause of disability and death in elderly patients.

_____ **2.** If you think an elderly person cannot hear what you are saying, you should shout directly into his or her ear to make sure you are understood.

_____ **3.** All elderly people are disabled in some way.

_____ **4.** You should make sure that elderly patients' eyeglasses are kept with them if possible.

_____ **5.** Most elderly people have trouble reading lips because all elderly people cannot see well.

_____ **6.** You should support elderly patients as they move because most are afraid of falling.

_____ **7.** When caring for patients with dementia, a kind and caring approach will make the patient more comfortable and will make your job easier.

_____ **8.** Loss of bowel or bladder control is common among the elderly and should not interfere with your care.

_____ **9.** If possible, you should send all medications to the hospital with elderly patients.

_____ **10.** Complex medical devices are not typically needed with patients who require long-term care.

_____ **11.** Many of the medical conditions that commonly occur in elderly patients can result in altered mental status.

_____ **12.** If you do not know sign language, the best way to communicate with a deaf person is to gesture or write a note.

_____ **13.** The best way to determine if a person is deaf is to ask "Can you hear me?" while turned away from the patient.

_____ **14.** Elderly patients may not take their medication as instructed.

_____ **15.** It is important for you to determine what types of medication a patient takes.

_____ **16.** During an emotional or medical crisis, the reassurance of your touch may be even more important to a blind person than to a person who can see.

_____ **17.** Today, most patients with serious chronic medical conditions are treated in hospitals or rehabilitation centers and, as a result, their lifespan has increased.

_____ **18.** Older patients are more likely to have a painful heart attack.

_____ **19.** Three types of mental problems seen frequently in older people are depression, suicidal thoughts, and dementia or Alzheimer disease.

_____ **20.** Depression is the most common psychiatric condition experienced by older adults.

_____ **21.** Elder abuse is generally easy to detect.

_____ **22.** One of the goals of a hospice is to provide pain relief through the use of needles and IVs.

_____ **23.** Living wills and do not resuscitate (DNR) orders are examples of advance directives.

_____ **24.** When caring for patients with dementia, it is important to speak clearly to them and use their names.

_____ **25.** Older men have a low rate of suicide in the United States.

Labeling

Label the following diagrams with the correct terms.

1. Simple Phrases in Sign Language

A. _____

B. _____

C. _____

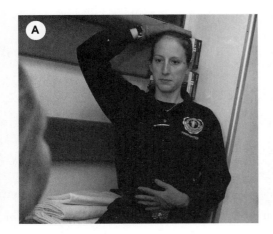

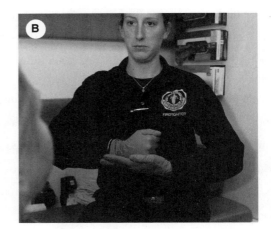

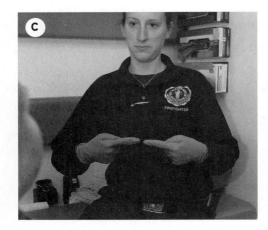

Crossword Puzzle

Use the clues in the column to complete the crossword puzzle.

Across

3. This term describes patients older than 65 years.
5. These animals may accompany blind patients.
6. _____ errors are a possible explanation for decreased vision or mental confusion in geriatric patients.
8. The muscles associated with respiration become weaker with aging, making it harder for elderly people to _____.
9. An action taken by a family member or caregiver that results in the physical, emotional, or sexual harm to a person older than 65 years.

Down

1. The most common type of dementia.
2. Rotated outward, such as in the case of a fractured hip.
4. This program provides end-of-life care to patients in their homes or in a special facility.
7. People with certain _____ ear disorders are more prone to poor balance and falls than the general population.

Critical Thinking

Fill-in-the-Blank

Read each item carefully and then complete the statement by filling in the missing words.

1. Elderly people often wear _____ clothing than younger people, even during warmer months.

2. Loss of bowel and _____ control occurs frequently in the geriatric population.

3. _____ _____ is an invisible disability.

4. _____ occur frequently in the geriatric population because the loss of bone density often results in osteoporosis.

5. Because elderly patients can have a variety of chronic conditions, many of them take a large number of _____ every day.

6. A(n) _____ is a health care program that brings together a variety of caregivers to provide physical, emotional, spiritual, social, and economic care for patients who have terminal illnesses.

7. _____ is a decrease in the density of bone that is common in postmenopausal women.

8. _____ _____ is a chronic degenerative disorder that attacks the brain and results in impaired memory, behavior, and thinking.

9. In a hip fracture, the injured leg is usually (but not always) _____ as compared with the other leg.

10. There are two major types of respiratory diseases: chronic and _____.

11. _____ is a common infectious disease in elderly patients.

12. _____ drain urine from the patient's bladder.

Fill-in-the-Table

Fill in the missing parts of the table.

Disabilities That May Occur With Age
• _____ loss or impairment
• Sight _____ or impairment
• Loss of _____
• _____ movements
• _____
• Senility
• Loss of _____ or _____ control

Short Answer

Complete this section with short written answers using the space provided.

1. Name three signs that would suggest that an elderly person has a broken hip.

_____

_____

2. List three important ways you can ease communication with older patients.

_____

_____

3. Name three signs of elder abuse.

_____

_____

4. List three factors that may contribute to suicide among older patients.

_____

_____

You Make the Call

The following scenarios provide an opportunity to explore the concerns associated with patient management. Read the scenarios and answer the questions to the best of your ability.

1. You arrive on the scene to find an 80-year-old woman complaining of dizziness. After assessing the situation, taking a patient history, and performing an examination, you find out that the patient has Alzheimer disease and may have overdosed on her medication. What should you do?

_____

_____

_____

2. You are dispatched to a local assisted living center for an 86-year-old woman who has fallen. The staff at the facility tell you the patient was walking down the hallway when she tripped and fell. The patient is alert but not oriented to her surroundings. You notice her left leg is shortened and externally rotated. What should you do?

_____

_____

_____

Lifting and Moving Patients

General Knowledge

Matching

Match each of the items in the left column to the appropriate definition in the right column.

_____ **1.** Arm-to-arm drag

_____ **2.** Blanket drag

_____ **3.** Clothes drag

_____ **4.** Fire fighter drag

_____ **5.** Log roll

_____ **6.** Recovery position

_____ **7.** Straddle lift

_____ **8.** Two-person walking assist

_____ **9.** Scoop stretcher

_____ **10.** Two-person extremity carry

A. A method used to place a patient on a backboard if there is not enough space to perform a log roll

B. Used to move a patient onto a long backboard

C. The rescuer grasps the patient's arms from behind; used to remove a patient from a hazardous place

D. A method of moving a patient without lifting or carrying him or her

E. Can be split into halves and applied to the patient from both sides

F. Helps an unconscious patient maintain an open airway

G. Used when the patient cannot bear his or her own weight

H. The rescuer encloses the patient in a blanket and drags the patient to safety

I. A method of carrying a patient out of tight quarters without equipment

J. The rescuer grasps the patient's clothes and moves the patient head first from the unsafe area

Multiple Choice

Read each item carefully and then select the one best response.

_____ **1.** A man who is lying on the ground next to his automobile must be moved. To protect the patient's spine, you should move him lengthwise with the:

  A. arm-to-arm drag.

  B. clothes or blanket drag.

  C. straddle lift or straddle slide.

  D. fire fighter drag.

_____ **2.** Which of the following can be used to successfully move a patient who is too heavy for a rescuer to lift or carry?

  A. Clothes or blanket drag

  B. Arm-to-arm drag

  C. Fire fighter drag

  D. All of the above

_____ **3.** Which drag provides some protection for the patient's head and neck?

  A. Clothes drag

  B. Blanket drag

  C. Arm-to-arm drag

  D. All of the above

_____ **4.** To perform a fire fighter drag:
    A. place the patient on a blanket or rug.
    B. tie the patient's hands around your neck.
    C. the patient must be wearing clothes that will not easily tear.
    D. all of the above.

_____ **5.** Moving a patient onto a long backboard:
    A. requires a team of four or five rescuers.
    B. can be performed with the use of log rolling.
    C. can be performed with the use of a straddle lift.
    D. all of the above.

_____ **6.** Log rolling a patient safely requires:
    A. a team of four rescuers.
    B. a long backboard.
    C. verbal commands.
    D. all of the above.

_____ **7.** The head and neck of a patient on a backboard:
    A. do not need further immobilization.
    B. may be immobilized with a short backboard.
    C. may be immobilized with foam blocks or a blanket roll.
    D. all of the above.

_____ **8.** A patient who is in a sitting position and has sustained possible head or spine injuries will probably need a:
    A. long backboard.
    B. short backboard device.
    C. scoop stretcher.
    D. stair chair.

_____ **9.** A scoop stretcher:
    A. is also called an orthopaedic stretcher.
    B. separates into halves.
    C. should not be used when there are head or spine injuries.
    D. all of the above.

_____ **10.** A patient should be transported on a backboard:
    A. in a face-up position.
    B. with the head and neck turned to one side.
    C. only when he or she is unconscious.
    D. all of the above.

_____ **11.** Transfer of a patient from a bed to a stretcher:
    A. uses the draw sheet method.
    B. requires the stretcher to be positioned perpendicular to the foot of the bed.
    C. should be used only when a patient is unconscious.
    D. all of the above.

_____ **12.** The two-person extremity carry:
    A. makes use of the patient's arms and legs.
    B. requires the use of equipment.
    C. allows the two rescuers to see each other.
    D. all of the above.

_____ **13.** The two-person seat carry:
    A. is used only for unconscious patients.
    B. requires the use of equipment.
    C. allows the two rescuers to see each other.
    D. all of the above.

_____ **14.** The cradle-in-arms carry:
    A. requires no equipment.
    B. can be used by one rescuer.
    C. is used to carry a child.
    D. all of the above.

_____ **15.** The two-person chair carry:
    A. requires the use of a folding chair.
    B. allows the patient to hold on to the chair.
    C. should not be used on stairways.
    D. all of the above.

_____ **16.** The pack-strap carry:
    A. requires the use of equipment.
    B. requires two rescuers.
    C. may use straps that are improvised.
    D. is a one-person carry.

_____ **17.** A portable moving device used to carry a patient in a sitting position is a:
    A. pack strap.
    B. portable stretcher.
    C. stair chair.
    D. reclining stretcher.

_____ **18.** Which of the following statements is false regarding wheeled ambulance stretchers?
    A. Wheeled ambulance stretchers are also called cots.
    B. If the loaded stretcher must be carried, it is best to use two people.
    C. Stretchers can be rolled or carried by two or four people.
    D. Each type of stretcher has its own set of levers and controls for raising and lowering the stretcher.

_____ **19.** After the short backboard device is applied:
    A. the patient is carefully placed on a long backboard.
    B. there is no need for further spine immobilization.
    C. release the straps to allow for better breathing.
    D. remove the cervical collar from the patient.

_____ **20.** Which of the following statements regarding the body mechanics of lifting is false?
    A. Use the strength of the large muscles in your legs to lift patients.
    B. Exercising good body mechanics helps to reduce the potential for injury when lifting.
    C. Lift while twisting your body for better body mechanics.
    D. Do not lift when your back is bent over a patient.

True/False

If you believe the statement to be more true than false, write the letter "T" in the space provided. If you believe the statement to be more false than true, write the letter "F."

_____ **1.** One rescuer alone should not attempt to remove a patient from any car involved in a motor vehicle crash.

_____ **2.** The use of the direct ground lift is discouraged because of the danger of back injuries to the rescuers.

_____ **3.** The direct ground lift is an appropriate lift for patients who have traumatic injuries.

_____ **4.** The direct ground lift requires the coordination of two rescuers.

_____ **5.** Walking assists for ambulatory patients should always involve two rescuers.

_____ **6.** The two rescuers completely support the patient when the two-person walking assist is used.

_____ **7.** Wheeled ambulance stretchers are also called cots.

_____ **8.** Wheeled ambulance stretchers require four rescuers to roll or carry it for safe transport.

_____ **9.** A portable stretcher may be required in areas that do not have adequate space for a wheeled ambulance stretcher.

_____ **10.** The frame of a portable stretcher is lighter weight than a wheeled ambulance stretcher.

_____ **11.** A stair chair is used to transport trauma patients up or down stairs.

_____ **12.** A long backboard is used for lifting or moving patients who have sustained trauma, especially back or neck injuries.

_____ **13.** Scoop stretchers are also called orthopaedic stretchers because they are used in cases of spine injuries.

_____ **14.** Improper initial treatment of patients who have sustained head or spine injuries can lead to paralysis.

_____ **15.** When used correctly, cervical collars will prevent all head and neck movement.

_____ **16.** A blanket roll or foam blocks may be used to immobilize the head and neck only if a cervical collar is not available.

_____ **17.** Both rigid and soft cervical collars provide sufficient support for trauma patients.

_____ **18.** A patient should be placed on a long backboard before a cervical collar is applied.

_____ **19.** A short backboard device is used instead of a long backboard when a patient is more comfortable in a sitting position.

_____ **20.** It is the responsibility of the EMR to apply the short backboard device before other medical personnel arrive at the scene of an incident.

_____ **21.** In confined spaces, the straddle lift can be used instead of the log-rolling technique.

_____ **22.** In a straddle slide, the patient is slid onto the backboard.

_____ **23.** A patient on a backboard should be strapped on at the shoulders, hips, and ankles to avoid sliding off the backboard.

_____ **24.** If a blanket roll is used to immobilize a patient's head and neck on a backboard, the roll should be secured with one of the straps found on the backboard.

_____ **25.** Immobilizing a patient on a long backboard ensures that the airway will remain open during transport.

_____ **26.** If you have to move a patient, you should try to move the patient as little as possible and in a way that will not cause further harm.

_____ **27.** If possible, you should wait to move a patient until additional help arrives on the scene.

_____ **28.** If you must move a patient, you should move the patient first and then begin treatment.

_____ **29.** As an EMR, you should concentrate on treatment. Let EMS personnel explain to the patient what is happening and move the patient if necessary.

_____ **30.** You must decide if there is enough room to perform CPR properly on a patient in cardiac arrest, and, if there is not, move the patient.

_____ **31.** There is no effective way to remove a patient from a vehicle by yourself without causing some movement to the patient's neck.

_____ **32.** The best way to move a patient from a vehicle when you are alone is to grasp the patient under the arms and cradle the head between your arms.

_____ **33.** If you must immediately remove a patient from a vehicle and two rescuers are present, the first rescuer can support the patient's head and neck, while the second rescuer moves the patient by lifting under the arms.

_____ **34.** Proper lifting requires the back to be as straight as possible and the leg muscles to do the work.

_____ **35.** As you are lifting, make sure you communicate with the other members of the lifting team.

Labeling

Label the following diagrams with the correct terms.

1. Carries and Drags

A. _____

B. _____

C. _____

D. _____

E. _____

F. _____

G. _____

H. _____

I. _____

J. _____

K. _____

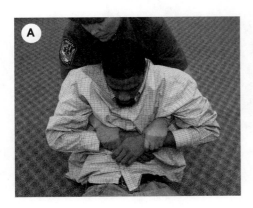

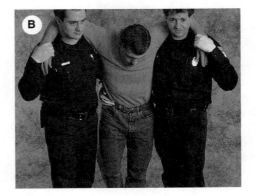

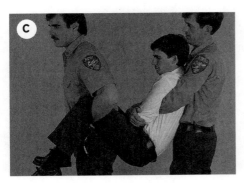

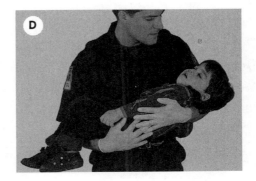

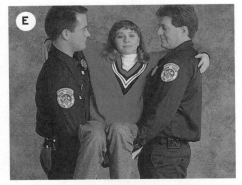

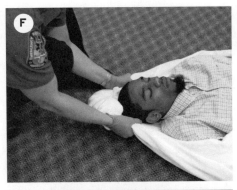

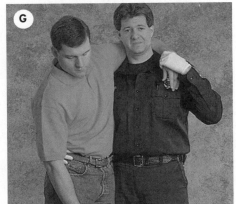

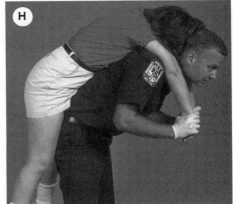

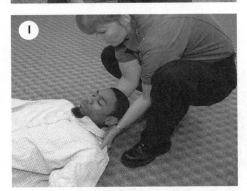

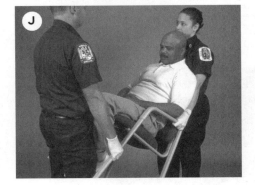

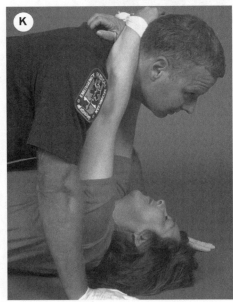

Crossword Puzzle

Use the clues in the column to complete the crossword puzzle.

Across

1. The _____ carry is a one-person carry that allows the rescuer to carry a patient while keeping one hand free.

3. The two-person _____ is a method of carrying a patient in which two rescuers use a chair to support the weight of the patient.

5. The one-person _____ is a method used if the patient is able to bear his or her own weight.

6. The two-person _____ is a method of carrying a patient in which two rescuers link arms behind the patient's back and under the patient's knees. This method requires no equipment.

7. A small portable device used for transporting a patient in a sitting position.

8. A method of placing a patient on a long backboard by straddling both the board and patient and sliding the patient onto the board.

Down

1. A lightweight nonwheeled device for transporting a patient; used in small spaces where the wheeled ambulance stretcher cannot be used.

2. The _____ carry is a one-rescuer patient movement technique used primarily for children; the patient is cradled in the hollow formed by the rescuer's arms and chest.

3. A neck brace that partially stabilizes the neck following injury.

4. The arms and legs.

Critical Thinking

Fill-in-the-Blank

Read each item carefully and then complete the statement by filling in the missing words.

1. The primary technique used to move a patient onto a long backboard is _____ _____.

2. The main purpose of backboards is to _____ the spine.

3. _____ _____ are used to prevent excess movement of the neck and head.

4. A(n) _____ stretcher or orthopaedic stretcher is a rigid device that is helpful in moving patients out of small spaces.

5. _____ cervical collars do not provide sufficient support for trauma patients.

6. When performing a log roll, the rescuer holding the patient's _____ should always give the commands to move the patient.

7. Because the log-rolling maneuver requires sufficient space for _____ rescuers, it is not always possible to perform it correctly.

8. A(n) _____ _____ is used when the wheeled stretcher cannot be moved into a small space.

9. The _____ _____ _____ is used to move a patient who is on the ground or the floor to an ambulance stretcher.

10. In an extreme emergency where a patient must be moved from a dangerous environment and a commercially prepared backboard is not available, you should _____.

Short Answer

Complete this section with short written answers using the space provided.

1. Name the two most common reasons why you would move a patient.

_____

_____

2. What should you do if you suspect that the patient has sustained trauma to the head or spine?

_____

_____

3. Why would the recovery position be used for an unconscious patient who has not sustained trauma?

_____

_____

4. Describe three situations that require moving a patient before emergency medical care is provided.

_____

_____

5. Name three pieces of equipment that EMS providers commonly use for lifting and moving patients.

_____

_____

6. Name six guidelines to keep in mind when deciding to move a patient.

_____

_____

7. List three items that can be used to improvise a backboard.

_____

_____

You Make the Call

The following scenarios provide an opportunity to explore the concerns associated with patient management. Read the scenarios and answer the questions to the best of your ability.

1. You and your partner are directed to an elderly man who lives in a house near a major fire. He says that he has a heart condition and gets out of breath after walking a few steps. What should you do?

_____

_____

_____

2. Your unit arrives at the scene of a motor vehicle crash involving a car striking a tree. The patient tells you she lost control of her vehicle after answering her cell phone. She complains of neck pain. There appears to be no life threats or safety concerns for you or the patient. Your partner calls for a transporting EMS unit. What should you do?

_____

_____

_____

Skills

Skill Drills

Test your knowledge of this skill by filling in the correct words in the photo caption.

Skill Drill 18-3: Four-Person Log Roll

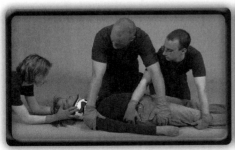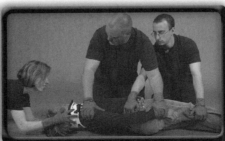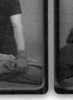

1. Rescuers get into position to _____ the patient.

2. Roll the patient onto his or her _____.

3. The fourth person slides the _____ toward the patient.

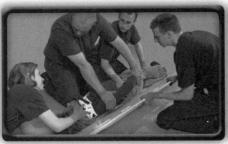

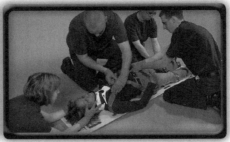

4. _____ the patient onto the backboard.

5. Center the patient on the backboard and _____ the patient before moving.

Skill Drill 18-5: Applying the Blanket Roll to Stabilize the Patient's Head and Neck

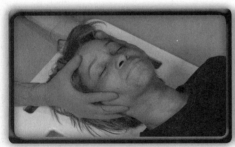

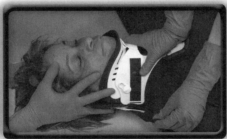

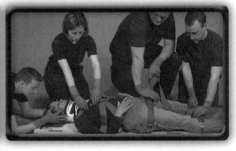

1. _____ the head.

2. Apply a(n) _____ _____.

3. Place the _____ around the backboard and patient.

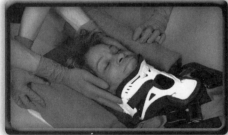

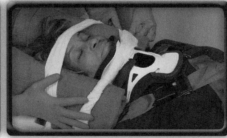

4. Insert the _____ _____ and roll each side of the blanket snugly against the _____ and shoulders.

5. Tie two _____ around the blanket roll, then two more around the blanket roll and backboard.

Transport Operations

General Knowledge

Matching

Match each phase of an EMS call in the left column to the appropriate activity(ies) in the right column.

_____ **1.** Preparation

_____ **2.** Dispatch

_____ **3.** Response to the scene

_____ **4.** Arrival at the scene

_____ **5.** Transferring care of the patient

_____ **6.** Postrun activities

A. Regularly inspect and maintain all emergency vehicles.

B. Notify your dispatcher or supervisor that you are ready for another call.

C. Drive safely to the scene of the emergency.

D. Perform a scene size-up.

E. Document all response activities.

F. Determine the number of patients.

G. Hand off a patient care report.

H. Receive dispatch information.

I. Determine the need for additional resources.

J. Use warning devices according to state laws and agency regulations.

Multiple Choice

Read each item carefully and then select the one best response.

_____ **1.** Which of the following is not performed in preparation for a call?

    A. Determine the best location to park your vehicle when arriving on scene.

    B. Follow a regular schedule to inspect and maintain all vehicles.

    C. Follow a checklist to ensure that everything is in working order.

    D. Check your stocked medical equipment on a scheduled basis.

_____ **2.** Dispatch information may be received through all of the following EXCEPT:

    A. a radio.

    B. a pager.

    C. an instant message.

    D. a computer terminal.

_____ **3.** When responding to the scene, you should:

    A. use warning lights because they guarantee you the right of way.

    B. be especially careful at intersections and railroad crossings.

    C. increase your speed on unpaved roads.

    D. drive offensively to avoid a potential crash.

_____ **4.** When you arrive at the scene, remember to place your vehicle:

    A. in a location that does not distract other drivers with your warning lights.

    B. as far away from the incident as possible.

    C. as close to the incident as possible.

    D. in a safe location to minimize the chance of injury.

_____ **5.** Which of the following is NOT part of the postrun activities?

    A. Documentation

    B. Cleaning your equipment

    C. Providing a brief report to the transporting EMS unit

    D. Replacing needed supplies

_____ **6.** All of the following are advantages of using helicopters in EMS EXCEPT:

    A. they can fly in all types of weather.

    B. they can quickly respond above traffic congestion.

    C. they typically carry specialized equipment.

    D. they can respond to wilderness areas.

_____ **7.** Most civilian helicopters need a landing zone of at least:

    A. 50′ × 50′.

    B. 100′ × 100′.

    C. 150′ × 150′.

    D. 200′ × 200′.

_____ **8.** When setting up a landing zone for a helicopter, you should:

    A. use flags to mark the perimeter.

    B. use fusees to mark the perimeter.

    C. turn on white lights and emergency lights to light up the scene.

    D. keep vehicles clear of the landing zone.

_____ **9.** All of the following are necessary precautions to take when loading a patient into a helicopter EXCEPT:

    A. securing loose clothing, sheets, and instruments.

    B. using eye protection.

    C. wearing reflective material on your clothes to make you more visible.

    D. approaching the helicopter from the front and only after the pilot or crew signals that it is safe.

_____ **10.** Which of the following statements regarding helicopter transport is false?

    A. Stand upright when approaching all helicopters.

    B. Hand off your patient care report to the flight crew away from the helicopter's noise.

    C. Certain safety precautions must be followed during the loading of a helicopter patient.

    D. You should check with your local helicopter service to see how you should secure and mark the perimeters of landing zones.

True/False

If you believe the statement to be more true than false, write the letter "T" in the space provided. If you believe the statement to be more false than true, write the letter "F."

_____ **1.** It is important to ensure that your emergency vehicles are ready to respond at all times.

_____ **2.** Most dispatch centers are part of a 9-1-1 system.

_____ **3.** You should still be able to respond to a scene properly without good dispatch information.

_____ **4.** Your first priority in responding to the scene is to get there quickly and safely.

_____ **5.** You should not waste time checking to make sure all responders are properly seated and secured in the emergency vehicle before responding to an incident.

_____ **6.** Warning lights and sirens guarantee you the right of way.

_____ **7.** When you arrive on scene, determine the number of patients and the need for additional resources.

_____ **8.** As more highly trained EMS personnel arrive on the scene, you will have to transfer care of the patient to them.

_____ **9.** The rotors of a helicopter can generate a "wash" equivalent to winds of 60 to 80 miles per hour.

_____ **10.** You should use white lights and flashing emergency lights when setting up a helicopter landing zone.

Crossword Puzzle

Use the clues in the column to complete the crossword puzzle.

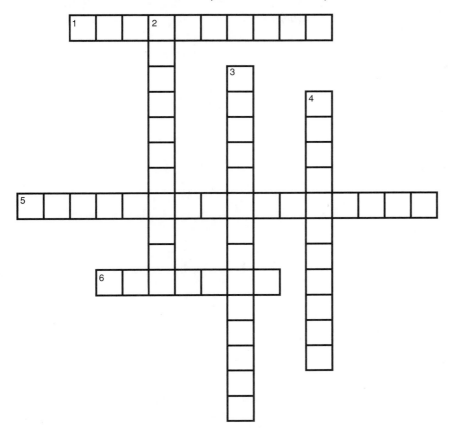

Across

1. Use of warning devices allows you to request _____, en route to an emergency scene.
5. A center that citizens can call to request emergency medical care.
6. _____ activities are performed by EMRs after patient care has been transferred to more highly trained EMS personnel.

Down

2. These emergency vehicles can respond more easily to wilderness areas but are limited by bad weather.
3. A(n) _____ kit contains patient examination, personal safety, resuscitation, bandaging and dressing, patient immobilization, extrication, and other equipment.
4. This area should be as flat as possible and free of debris that could become airborne in the 60-mph winds generated by a helicopter.

Critical Thinking

Fill-in-the-Blank

Read each item carefully and then complete the statement by filling in the missing words.

1. Most _____ _____ are responsible for dispatching fire, police, and EMS.

2. During response to the scene, keep all equipment secured so it does not become a(n) _____ in the event of a sudden stop or crash.

3. Control the flow of traffic to ensure safety to rescuers, patients, and _____.

4. _____ can provide lifesaving transport for patients with serious injuries to an appropriate medical facility.

5. _____ are red signal flares, and should not be used to mark a landing zone because they create a fire hazard.

Short Answer

Complete this section with short written answers using the space provided.

1. List six safety steps you should follow when working around an EMS helicopter.

_____

_____

2. What are the several "DO NOTs" associated with helicopters?

_____

_____

You Make the Call

The following scenarios provide an opportunity to explore the concerns associated with patient management. Read the scenarios and answer the questions to the best of your ability.

1. You arrive at the scene of a motor vehicle crash involving three vehicles. There are multiple patients with injuries. As several other EMRs are triaging patients, one of the responders yells for you to dispatch a helicopter and set up a landing zone. How are you going to handle this?

_____

_____

_____

2. You are the first to arrive at an intersection where a motor vehicle crash has just taken place. There is a large crowd of people standing around, and traffic seems to be stopped in both directions. You notice large debris in the roadway from the vehicles and see fluids leaking as well. How are you going to handle this?

_____

_____

_____

Vehicle Extrication and Special Rescue

General Knowledge

Matching

Match each of the items in the left column to the appropriate definition in the right column.

_____ **1.** Decompression sickness

_____ **2.** Flotation device

_____ **3.** Reach-throw-row-go

_____ **4.** Riptides

_____ **5.** Air embolism

_____ **6.** Chocking

_____ **7.** Fusees

_____ **8.** Extrication

_____ **9.** Tempered glass

_____ **10.** Hazardous materials

A. Unusually strong surface currents flowing outward from a seashore that can carry swimmers out to sea

B. Removal from a difficult situation or position

C. Toxic, poisonous, radioactive, flammable, or explosive substances

D. Condition seen in divers in which gas, especially nitrogen, forms bubbles in blood vessels, obstructing them

E. Breaks into small pieces when hit with a sharp, pointed object

F. A bubble of air obstructing a blood vessel

G. Warning devices or flares that burn with a red color

H. A piece of wood or metal placed in front of or behind a wheel

I. Four-step reminder of the sequence of actions that should be taken in water rescue situations

J. Includes life rings and life buoys

Multiple Choice

Read each item carefully and then select the one best response.

_____ **1.** In a water rescue, you should enter the water only if you:

A. are sure the person will not panic and drag you under.

B. do not have a flotation device available.

C. know the struggling person cannot swim.

D. are a capable swimmer trained in lifesaving techniques.

_____ **2.** The best way to turn an unresponsive patient who is face down in the water is to:

A. lift up on the patient's chest with both hands.

B. hold the patient by both shoulders and then push up on one shoulder and down on the other.

C. pull the patient's head up out of the water.

D. turn the patient as a unit while stabilizing the head and neck.

_____ **3.** If you must rescue someone who has fallen through ice, you should tie a rope around your waist and secure it to a sturdy object on shore. Next, you should:

A. crawl out to the victim.

B. walk quickly out to the victim.

C. push yourself across the ice on your stomach.

D. slowly walk across the ice.

4. If you are called to rescue people from a motor vehicle on the ice, you should ask them to open the vehicle's doors so that:
   A. the vehicle will sink more slowly if the ice breaks.
   B. the windows will be less likely to break and cause injury to the vehicle's occupants.
   C. you will be able to see the people in the vehicle more clearly.
   D. the door jams won't freeze.

5. Which of the following is false regarding the "throw" step of the water rescue sequence?
   A. If you cannot reach the person, throw something.
   B. Only Coast-Guard-approved, life-saving devices should be used.
   C. A spare tire can support several people.
   D. Rescuers should have training before using a rescue throw bag.

6. All of the following are part of scuba gear EXCEPT:
   A. a wetsuit.
   B. a regulator.
   C. a mouthpiece and face mask.
   D. an air tank.

7. The two specialized injuries associated with diving are:
   A. air embolism and decompression sickness.
   B. air embolism and suffocation.
   C. decompression sickness and hyperventilation.
   D. decompression sickness and suffocation.

8. Signs and symptoms of an air bubble affecting the brain or spinal cord may be similar to those of:
   A. a heart attack.
   B. a stroke.
   C. flu.
   D. choking.

9. Signs and symptoms of a diving accident include all of the following EXCEPT:
   A. difficulty speaking.
   B. difficulty breathing.
   C. abdominal pain.
   D. vomiting.

10. During an ice rescue, you may be at risk for:
   A. air embolism.
   B. hyperthermia.
   C. hypothermia.
   D. the bends.

11. Because of the large numbers of people being transported by buses:
   A. there is an increased risk for terrorist activity in urban areas.
   B. there is significant potential for bus crashes to occur in any community.
   C. there is potential for fewer injuries annually due to more cars on the roadways.
   D. there is an increased risk for illnesses related to pollution.

12. As you approach a motor vehicle crash scene, but before you exit your vehicle:
   A. immediately request assistance.
   B. determine the mechanism of injury.
   C. assess for possible routes of extrication.
   D. get an overview of the entire incident.

_____ **13.** Which of the following is true when dealing with infectious diseases during a rescue operation?

    A. Follow standard precautions at all motor vehicle crashes.

    B. Latex gloves are sufficient protection from blood splatters.

    C. Leather gloves provide effective protection from bodily fluids.

    D. If sharp glass or metal is present, use face protection.

_____ **14.** All of the following are true regarding motor vehicle batteries EXCEPT:

    A. batteries are hazardous, and you must avoid contact with them.

    B. you should not attempt to disconnect a battery unless you are trained.

    C. you could be injured by a short circuit, explosion, or contact with battery acid.

    D. you should leave the engine running to reduce the possibility of a short circuit.

_____ **15.** Postimpact fires in motor vehicle crashes are often caused by:

    A. a leaking gas tank.

    B. excessive heat from the engine compartment.

    C. an electrical short circuit.

    D. airbag deployment.

_____ **16.** If you must break a window to open a door in a motor vehicle:

    A. always break one on the passenger's side.

    B. always break the windshield.

    C. try to break one that is farthest from the patient.

    D. try to break one that is on the same side as the patient.

_____ **17.** Which of the following statements regarding air bags is false?

    A. You should always be alert for undeployed air bags when entering a vehicle.

    B. The side-mounted air bag does not pose a risk to rescuers.

    C. You should avoid getting in front of an undeployed air bag.

    D. Air bags are mounted in the steering wheel on the driver's side and in the dashboard on the passenger's side.

_____ **18.** What is the fourth step in the extrication process?

    A. Patient removal

    B. Patient disentanglement

    C. Initial emergency care

    D. Access to patient

_____ **19.** Which of the following is not a hazard typically found on a farm?

    A. Poisonous plants

    B. Pesticides

    C. Herbicides

    D. Machines

_____ **20.** What are the two deadly hazards associated with rescue situations involving confined space?

    A. Respiratory emergencies and structural collapse

    B. Respiratory emergencies and heart attack

    C. Heart attack and structural collapse

    D. Heart attack and spinal trauma

True/False

If you believe the statement to be more true than false, write the letter "T" in the space provided. If you believe the statement to be more false than true, write the letter "F."

_____ **1.** A person who has sustained a diving injury may have signs and symptoms similar to those of a stroke.

_____ **2.** It is not always necessary to turn patients who are face down in the water face up.

_____ **3.** You should use the jaw-thrust maneuver to open the airway of a patient in the water, but the head should be kept in a neutral position.

_____ **4.** A patient who you believe has a spinal cord injury should be removed from the water on something that will provide support for the back.

_____ **5.** Neck pain and numbness or tingling in the arms or legs are signs of spinal cord injury in a responsive patient needing rescue from the water.

_____ **6.** If no rigid support is available to move an unresponsive person from the water, you and one other rescuer can provide adequate support to lift the person out of the water.

_____ **7.** In a bus rescue, patients and equipment should be passed through the same window for maximum efficiency and speed.

_____ **8.** Reach, throw, row, and go are rescue steps used primarily when it is too cold for the rescuer to enter the water.

_____ **9.** Do not try to break and enter through the windshield of a vehicle because it is made of plastic-laminated glass.

_____ **10.** If you cannot gain access to a vehicle, you must do what you can to assist the patients.

_____ **11.** Silos should always be treated as hazardous confined spaces.

_____ **12.** Rescue situations involving confined spaces typically have one deadly hazard.

_____ **13.** If your water rescue patient has experienced cardiac arrest, you should immediately begin CPR.

_____ **14.** You should treat a patient who is unconscious in the water as if a spinal cord injury were present.

_____ **15.** You should remove a patient from the water before beginning rescue breathing.

_____ **16.** In diving accidents, pink or bloody froth coming from the mouth may be a sign of a collapsed lung.

_____ **17.** In diving accidents, severe abdominal pain may be a sign of recompression.

_____ **18.** In a bus collision involving multiple casualties, EMRs can be expected to handle the command functions.

_____ **19.** Confined spaces are structures that are designed to keep something in or out.

_____ **20.** Rescue situations involving confined spaces are hazardous because there may be insufficient oxygen to support life or a poisonous gas may be present.

_____ **21.** You should park your vehicle at a scene so that it protects the scene and warns oncoming traffic to avoid the crash site.

_____ **22.** A rope or police/fire barrier tape is usually not very effective at establishing an off-limits area.

_____ **23.** You should treat all downed wires as if they are charged until you receive specific clearance from the electric company.

_____ **24.** Assume that every vehicle involved in a crash is unstable.

_____ **25.** An upside-down vehicle is relatively unstable.

Crossword Puzzle

Use the clues in the column to complete the crossword puzzle.

Across

3. Farm rescues require EMRs to follow the seven steps of _____.

5. A water rescue device consisting of a small cloth bag and a waterproof rope used for rescuing people from the water.

7. Be especially alert for these hazards after a storm that has blown down trees and tree limbs.

8. This type of fire occurs when the gas tank ruptures during a motor vehicle crash.

Down

1. Wooden _____ describes 2″ × 4″ or 4″ × 4″ boards used for stabilization or bracing.

2. This type of spill is a fire hazard and is common during motor vehicle crashes.

4. A condition seen in divers in which gas, especially nitrogen, forms bubbles in blood vessels, obstructing them; also known as decompression sickness.

6. A concept of emergency patient care that attempts to place a trauma patient into definitive medical care in the shortest period of time to achieve the best possible outcome.

9. As soon as you arrive at the scene of an ice rescue, visually _____ the location where the person was last seen.

Critical Thinking

Fill-in-the-Blank
Read each item carefully and then complete the statement by filling in the missing words.

1. At a swimming pool, dock, or supervised beach, a(n) _____ device may be available.

2. The four steps of a water rescue are reach, throw, _____, and go.

3. If you are involved in a water rescue situation, your primary concerns for the patient must be to open a(n) _____, establish breathing and circulation, and stabilize spinal cord injuries.

4. When turning a patient in the water, make sure to stabilize the _____ and _____.

5. Two specialized injuries are associated with diving: _____ embolism and _____ _____.

6. In confined space rescues, you must be careful of hazards, including insufficient _____ and danger of collapse.

7. In farm rescues, reporting of the emergency may be _____.

8. _____ are unusually strong surface currents flowing outward from the seashore that can carry swimmers out to sea.

9. When you see a person struggling in the water, your first impulse may be to _____ in to assist, but this is a mistake.

10. If a swimmer has experienced _____ _____, quickly stabilize the head and neck, and remove the patient from the water.

11. Assume that every vehicle involved in a crash is _____, unless you have manually _____ it.

12. When providing initial emergency care during vehicle extrication, leave the patients in the vehicle unless it is on _____ or they are otherwise in immediate danger.

13. The concept of the _____ _____ means that the less time spent at the scene with a seriously injured patient, the better.

14. The _____ route must be large enough to permit the safe removal of a packaged patient.

15. The third step in the extrication process is to _____ _____ to the patients.

Short Answer
Complete this section with short written answers using the space provided.

1. List, in order, the four steps you should follow when attempting a water or ice rescue.

_____

_____

2. Name three common signs or symptoms of diving injuries.

_____

_____

3. List five confined spaces where you might encounter as an EMR.

_____

_____

4. What are the two deadly hazards you may face when involved with a confined space rescue?

_____

_____

5. What are the seven steps of extrication?

_____

_____

You Make the Call

The following scenarios provide an opportunity to explore the concerns associated with patient management. Read the scenarios and answer the questions to the best of your ability.

1. You are dispatched to a farm for the report of an injured person. When you arrive, you find the patient in a farm silo. He has fallen about 15 feet from the top of the silo and appears to be unconscious. A coworker of the patient says he thinks he had a heart attack. What should you do?

_____

_____

_____

2. You are the first unit to arrive at the scene of a motor vehicle crash. As you approach the scene, you notice that the engine compartment of one of the involved vehicles is on fire and that two passengers are trapped inside. What should you do?

_____

_____

_____

Skills

Skill Drills

Test your knowledge of this skill by filling in the correct words in the photo caption.

Skill Drill 20-1: Accessing the Vehicle Through the Window

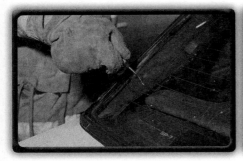 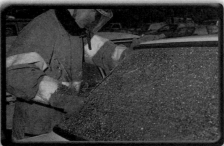

1. Place the spring-loaded center punch at the _____ corner of the _____.

2. Press the center punch to _____ the window.

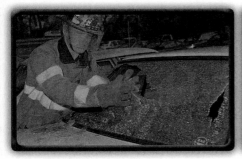 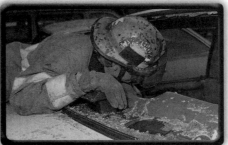

3. Remove the _____ to the outside.

4. Enter the _____ through the _____.

Skill Drill 20-3: Turning a Patient in the Water

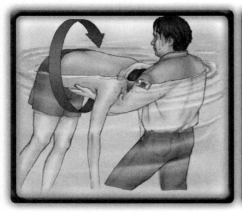 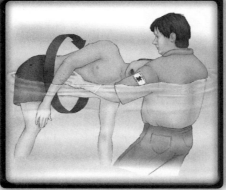 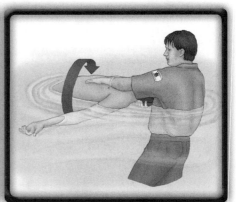

1. Support the _____ and _____ with one hand. Place your other hand on the _____ of the patient.

2. Carefully turn the patient as a(n) _____.

3. Stabilize the patient's _____ and _____.

Incident Management

General Knowledge

Matching

Match each of the items in the left column to the appropriate definition in the right column.

_____ 1. Blister agents

_____ 2. Biologic agents

_____ 3. Chemical agents

_____ 4. Nerve agents

_____ 5. Metabolic agents

_____ 6. Pulmonary agents

_____ 7. Decontamination

_____ 8. Terrorism

_____ 9. Warm zone

_____ 10. Radiation

_____ 11. Hot zone

_____ 12. Incendiary device

_____ 13. Cold zone

_____ 14. Dirty bomb

_____ 15. Triage

A. Substances that are intended to produce injury or death by disrupting chemical reactions at the cellular level

B. An explosive device designed to disperse radioactive material over a wide area

C. The process of reducing or preventing the spread of contaminants at a hazardous materials event

D. Toxic substances that attack the central nervous system

E. Chemicals that cause the skin to blister

F. The control area that contains the command post and other support functions needed in the incident

G. The control area where personnel and equipment decontamination takes place

H. Disease-causing bacteria or viruses that might be used by terrorists to intentionally cause epidemics of disease

I. An appliance designed to start fires

J. The sorting of patients into groups according to the severity of their injuries

K. Substances that produce respiratory distress or illness

L. Compounds that can be used by terrorists to inflict harm

M. A contaminated area

N. A systematic use of violence to intimidate or to achieve a goal

O. The electromagnetic energy that is released from radioactive material

Multiple Choice

Read each item carefully and then select the one best response.

_____ 1. Which of the following symptoms could be caused by a nerve agent?

A. Urination

B. Excessive tearing

C. Gastric upset

D. All of the above

_____ 2. When arriving on the scene of a suspected terrorist event, your first responsibility is to:

A. assess scene safety.

B. set up the incident command system.

C. start triage.

D. request additional resources.

_____ **3.** Safety considerations for EMRs dealing with incidents involving radiation include:
  A. staying away from the source of radiation until specially trained teams arrive.
  B. using standard precautions.
  C. remaining downwind of the blast site.
  D. all of the above.

_____ **4.** Which of the following is an example of terrorism?
  A. Bombing of an abortion clinic
  B. Intimidating national event where property was damaged but no lives were lost
  C. Attacks on the World Trade Center and the Pentagon on September 11, 2001
  D. All of the above

_____ **5.** Infrastructure that may be affected by weapons of mass destruction includes:
  A. bridges and tunnels.
  B. airports and seaports.
  C. electrical power plants.
  D. all of the above.

_____ **6.** Shortness of breath, flushed skin, rapid heartbeat, seizures, coma, and cardiac arrest are possible symptoms of exposure to:
  A. insecticides.
  B. cyanides.
  C. blister agents.
  D. radiation.

_____ **7.** SLUDGE is an acronym to help remember:
  A. common hazardous materials.
  B. important safety considerations.
  C. symptoms of exposure to organophosphate insecticides or nerve agents.
  D. steps in response to suspected terrorist events.

_____ **8.** Common targets of terrorists include all of the following EXCEPT:
  A. farms.
  B. undeveloped land.
  C. housing developments.
  D. churches.

_____ **9.** Common signs of low levels of exposure to radiation include:
  A. hair loss.
  B. cancer.
  C. vomiting.
  D. death.

_____ **10.** Which of the following is not addressed within the scope of NIMS?
  A. Command and Management
  B. Family Support
  C. Resource Management
  D. Preparedness

_____ **11.** Which of the following are considered hazardous materials?

    A. Toxins

    B. Poisons

    C. Flammable substances

    D. All of the above

_____ **12.** Federal law requires that all vehicles containing certain quantities of hazardous materials:

    A. drive under the posted speed limits.

    B. display a hazardous materials placard.

    C. drive with their hazard lights flashing at all times.

    D. display a permit in the passenger window.

_____ **13.** Your goal at a multiple-casualty incident is to:

    A. provide the greatest medical benefit for the greatest number of people.

    B. assume command and prevent chaos.

    C. treat as many patients as possible in the shortest amount of time.

    D. treat only those who are likely to survive.

_____ **14.** Your first step when arriving at the scene of a mass-casualty incident is to:

    A. contact the communications center to declare a disaster.

    B. begin immediate triage.

    C. make a visual assessment of the entire scene.

    D. establish incident command according to NIMS guidelines.

_____ **15.** Which of the following statements regarding triage is false?

    A. It is essential that you make specific diagnoses before you categorize patients.

    B. Avoid spending undue time treating the first or second patient you see.

    C. You must identify and separate patients rapidly, according to the severity of their injuries and their need for treatment.

    D. You should not stop during the triage process, except to correct airway and severe bleeding problems quickly.

_____ **16.** All of the following are part of the levels of triage EXCEPT:

    A. immediate care.

    B. intermediate care.

    C. urgent care.

    D. delayed care.

_____ **17.** A patient at a mass-casualty scene presents with severe chest trauma, a respiratory rate greater than 30 times a minutes, and is pale and sweaty. What is the triage category for this patient?

    A. Red

    B. Yellow

    C. Green

    D. Black

_____ **18.** Any patient that is able to walk during the initial triage is categorized as:

    A. red.

    B. yellow.

    C. green.

    D. black.

_____ **19.** The second part of the triage assessment is:

    A. ability to walk.

    B. respirations.

    C. circulation.

    D. injuries.

_____ **20.** The person who is ultimately in charge of the rescue operation at an incident is the:

    A. administrative director.

    B. logistics director.

    C. EMS operations supervisor.

    D. incident commander.

_____ **21.** The National Incident Management System (NIMS) was developed by the:

    A. Federal Emergency Management Agency.

    B. US Department of Homeland Security.

    C. National Highway and Transportation Safety Administration.

    D. US Department of Transportation.

_____ **22.** As an EMR, your role falls within the _____ category of NIMS.

    A. Command and Management

    B. Preparedness

    C. Resource Management

    D. Supporting Technologies

True/False

If you believe the statement to be more true than false, write the letter "T" in the space provided. If you believe the statement to be more false than true, write the letter "F."

_____ **1.** Radiation is a hidden hazard that is similar to electricity.

_____ **2.** Unless there was a warning issued about such an event, rescuers might not know about the presence of radiation.

_____ **3.** Explosives are sometimes used to start fires.

_____ **4.** When vapors of blistering agents are inhaled, they can cause burns in the digestive system.

_____ **5.** Chlorine is an example of a pulmonary agent.

_____ **6.** Metabolic agents are typically only found in textile mills.

_____ **7.** Your top priority at a hazardous materials incident is to identify exposed patients.

_____ **8.** The first step in START is to tell all the people who can get up and walk to move to a specific area.

_____ **9.** Injured patients typically remain in the same condition.

_____ **10.** When weapons of mass destruction have been used, it is generally safe to enter where the event has occurred.

Crossword Puzzle

Use the clues in the column to complete the crossword puzzle.

Across

4. A system of casualty sorting using simple triage and rapid treatment.

8. Chemicals that are formulated to kill insects, but can intentionally or accidentally cause injury or death to humans.

9. The structure for managing an emergency incident, which may require a response from many different agencies; designed to provide efficient and effective management from initial response through recovery.

10. _____ materials are toxic, poisonous, radioactive, flammable, or explosive and can cause injury or death from exposure.

11. A contaminated area.

Down

1. The time from exposure to a disease organism to the time the person begins to show symptoms of the disease.

2. The sorting of patients for treatment and transportation.

3. _____ incidents are accidents or situations involving more patients than you can handle with the initial resources available.

5. A set of people, procedures, and equipment designed to improve emergency response operations at situations of all types and complexities.

6. Any agent designed to bring about mass death, casualties, and/or massive damage to property and infrastructure (eg, bridges, tunnels, airports, electrical power plants, seaports).

7. Substances that release energy in a sudden and uncontrolled manner when detonated.

Critical Thinking

Fill-in-the-Blank

Read each item carefully and then complete the statement by filling in the missing words.

1. A(n) _____ of _____ _____ is any agent designed to bring about mass death, casualties, and/or massive damage to property and infrastructure.

2. An agent used to produce a concussion that destroys property and inflicts injury and death is a(n) _____.

3. A personal _____ measures the amount of radioactive exposure received by an individual.

4. Anthrax and smallpox are examples of _____ agents.

5. A(n) _____ period is the time from a person's exposure to a disease organism to the time symptoms appear.

6. The _____ triage system is designed to help you find the most seriously injured patients.

7. The _____ _____ _____ lists the most common hazardous materials, their four-digit identification numbers, and the proper emergency actions to control the scene.

8. A(n) _____ _____ is a contaminated area where people can be exposed to sharp metal edges, broken glass, toxic substances, lethal rays, or ignition or explosion of hazardous materials.

9. Priority Two or _____ _____ patients are identified with a yellow tag.

10. A dead patient gets a(n) _____ or _____ tag during the triage process.

Short Answer

Complete this section with short written answers using the space provided.

1. List the five categories of chemical agents.

_____

_____

2. Name three symptoms of exposure to an organophosphate insecticide or nerve agent.

_____

_____

3. Name the three common signs of acute radiation sickness with low exposure.

_____

_____

4. Identify three locations where radiation is commonly used.

_____

_____

5. What are the signs and symptoms of cyanide exposure?

_____

_____

6. What are the key points to communicate when declaring a disaster?

_____

_____

7. What does the acronym START stand for?

_____

_____

8. What are the six major areas within the scope of NIMS?

_____

_____

You Make the Call

The following scenarios provide an opportunity to explore the concerns associated with patient management. Read the scenarios and answer the questions to the best of your ability.

1. You respond to a frantic call from dispatch stating that a white powder has been found in the post office downtown. You respond to the call within 2 minutes of initial dispatch and arrive to find several employees screaming and running around with small particles of white powder on their clothes. What should you do?

_____

_____

_____

2. You are the first to arrive at a scene involving a motor vehicle crash between two cars and a bus. There are multiple people walking around with obvious injuries. The bus is on its side and there is smoke coming from the engine compartment. What should you do?

_____

_____

_____

Chapter 1: EMS Systems

General Knowledge

Matching

1. F (page 7)
2. G (page 7)
3. E (page 7)
4. C (page 7)
5. B (page 7)
6. A (page 7)
7. D (page 7)
8. H (page 5)

Multiple Choice

1. D (page 15)
2. B (page 15)
3. D (page 12)
4. D (page 10)
5. A (page 5)
6. C (page 7)
7. A (page 7)
8. A (page 8)
9. C (pages 8–9)
10. A (page 9)
11. C (page 9)
12. A (page 9)
13. D (page 12)
14. C (page 13)
15. D (page 13)
16. C (page 15)
17. C (page 5)
18. B (page 15)
19. C (page 13)
20. D (pages 10–11)
21. C (page 8)
22. B (page 8)
23. C (page 8)

True/False

1. T (page 5)
2. F (page 13)
3. T (page 11)
4. T (page 9)
5. F (pages 5–6)
6. F (page 7)
7. T (page 12)
8. T (page 15)
9. F (page 13)
10. T (page 15)
11. F (page 15)
12. F (page 5)
13. F (page 10)
14. F (pages 10–11)
15. T (page 5)
16. F (page 6)
17. F (page 6)
18. F (page 6)
19. T (page 12)
20. T (page 13)

Crossword Puzzle

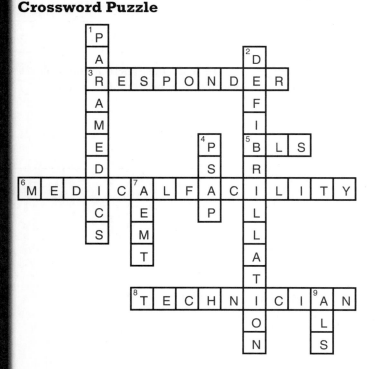

Critical Thinking

Fill-in-the-Blank

1. additional hazard (page 12)
2. confidential (page 13)
3. improvise; assist (pages 10–11)
4. law enforcement (page 6)
5. emergency response communications center; public safety answering point (page 5)

Short Answer

1. 1. Regulation and policy
   2. Resource management
   3. Human resources and training
   4. Transportation equipment and systems
   5. Medical and support facilities
   6. Communications systems
   7. Public information and education
   8. Medical direction
   9. Trauma system and development
   10. Evaluation (pages 8–9)
2. 1. First response
   2. EMS response
   3. Hospital care (pages 6–7)
3. Any three of the following:
   - Condition of the patient when found
   - Patient description of injury and/or illness
   - Initial and later vital signs
   - Treatment you gave the patient
   - Agency and personnel that took over treatment
   - Any other helpful facts (page 13)
4. 1. Know what you should not do.
   2. Know how to use your EMR life support kit.
   3. Know how to improvise.
   4. Know how to assist other EMS providers. (pages 10–11)
5. Medical oversight ensures that the patient receives appropriate medical treatment. (page 15)
6. Any five of the following:
   - Flashlight
   - Gloves
   - Face masks
   - Hand sanitizer
   - Mouth-to-mask resuscitation device
   - Portable hand-powered suction device
   - Oral airways
   - Nasal airways
   - Gauze strips or pads
   - Universal trauma dressings
   - Occlusive dressings
   - Gauze rolls
   - Bandages
   - Adhesive tape
   - Burn sheet
   - Cervical collars
   - Splints
   - Spring-loaded center punch
   - Heavy leather gloves
   - Blankets
   - Cold packs
   - Scissors
   - Protective clothing (helmet, eye protection, EMS jacket)
   - Reflective vest
   - Fire extinguisher
   - *Emergency Response Guidebook*
   - Flares
   - Binoculars (page 11)
7. 1. Safety
   2. Effectiveness
   3. Patient-centeredness
   4. Timeliness
   5. Efficiency
   6. Equitability (page 15)

You Make the Call

1. Your answer should include the following steps and information:
   - Communicate with the paramedics.
   - Inform the paramedics of what you have discovered about the patient's condition and what treatment you have provided.
   - Be prepared to assist the paramedics.
   - Prepare documentation, including your observations about the scene, the patient's condition, and the treatment you provided. (page 13)

Chapter 2: Workforce Safety and Wellness

General Knowledge

Matching

1. D (page 22)
2. G (page 28)
3. C (page 22)
4. F (page 27)
5. A (page 22)
6. E (page 22)
7. B (page 22)

Multiple Choice

1. C (pages 23–25)
2. D (pages 27–28)
3. C (page 25)
4. B (page 28)
5. D (page 22)
6. B (page 23)
7. B (page 23)
8. D (page 25)
9. A (page 22)
10. C (page 22)
11. B (page 22)
12. D (page 27)
13. A (pages 27–28)
14. A (page 27)
15. C (page 28)
16. D (page 28)
17. D (pages 28–29)
18. D (page 30)
19. A (pages 30–31)
20. D (page 32)
21. D (page 31)
22. B (pages 32–33)
23. B (page 32)
24. D (page 32)
25. C (page 32)

True/False

1. F (page 21)
2. F (page 21)
3. T (page 23)
4. F (page 25)
5. T (page 24)
6. F (page 25)
7. T (page 23)
8. F (pages 28–29)
9. F (page 28)
10. F (page 27)
11. T (page 34)
12. F (page 25)
13. F (pages 27–28)
14. T (page 28)
15. F (page 28)
16. T (page 28)
17. T (pages 27–28)
18. F (page 29)
19. F (page 32)
20. T (page 32)
21. F (page 33)
22. T (page 33)
23. T (page 28)
24. F (page 28)
25. T (page 30)
26. F (page 28)

Crossword Puzzle

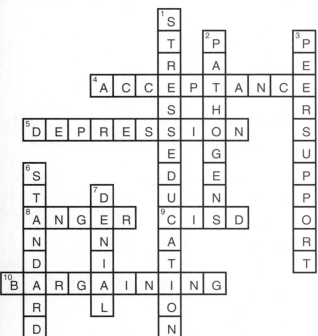

Critical Thinking

Fill-in-the-Blank

1. reducing (pages 23–25)
2. 8 (page 23)
3. Preincident (page 25)
4. peer (page 25)
5. critical incident stress debriefing (page 25)

6. Vehicle crashes (page 31)
7. Unstable (page 32)
8. invisible; current; qualified (page 32)
9. sharp objects (page 33)
10. changed; controlled (page 33)

Short Answer

1. Calls involving any three of the following:
   - A patient who reminds you of a family member
   - Very young or old patients
   - Critical patients
   - Death
   - Unusual danger
   - Violence
   - Unusual sights, smells, or sounds
   - Mass-casualty situations (page 21)

2. Any five of the following:
   - Irritability
   - Inability to concentrate
   - Change in normal disposition
   - Difficulty in sleeping or nightmares
   - Anxiety
   - Indecisiveness
   - Guilt
   - Loss of appetite
   - Loss of interest in sexual relations
   - Loss of interest in work
   - Isolation
   - Feelings of hopelessness
   - Alcohol or drug misuse or abuse
   - Physical symptoms (page 23)

3. 1. Always wear approved latex or nitrile gloves when handling patients, and change gloves after contact with each patient.
   2. Always wear a protective mask, eyewear, or a face shield when you anticipate that blood or other bodily fluids may splatter.
   3. Wash your hands and other skin surfaces immediately and thoroughly with soap and water if they become contaminated, change contaminated clothing, and wash exposed skin thoroughly.
   4. Do not recap, cut, or bend used needles. Place them directly in a puncture-resistant container designed for "sharps."
   5. Use a face shield, pocket mask, or other airway adjunct when providing resuscitation. (pages 28–29)

4. Any three of the following:
   - Protect the area from traffic hazards.
   - Check that emergency warning lights are operating correctly.
   - Carefully exit the vehicle.
   - Wear an approved safety vest.
   - Leave room for other arriving vehicles.
   - Protect the scene from further accidents. (page 31)

5. 1. Water rescue
   2. Ice rescue
   3. Confined space or below-grade rescue
   4. Terrorism
   5. Mass-casualty incidents (page 34)

6. Any five of the following:
   - Infectious diseases
   - Traffic
   - Crime or violence
   - Crowds
   - Electrical hazards
   - Fire
   - Hazardous materials
   - Unstable objects
   - Sharp objects
   - Animals
   - Environmental conditions
   - Special rescue situations (pages 27, 32–34)

7. 1. Denial
   2. Anger
   3. Bargaining
   4. Depression
   5. Acceptance (page 22)

You Make the Call

1. Your answer should include the following steps and information:

- Consider waiting at a safe distance for additional law enforcement if you have any doubts about scene safety.
- Approach carefully, making sure the scene is secure before entering.
- Take a mental picture of the scene and avoid disturbing anything unless it is necessary to move objects to provide patient care.
- Perform a patient assessment and treat your patient. (page 32)

2. Your answer should include the following steps and information:

- This patient has likely acquired a communicable illness, possibly tuberculosis. First, protect yourself and follow standard precautions. Place a mask over your face, preferably a high-efficiency particulate air (HEPA) respirator.
- Provide high-flow oxygen to the patient via a nonrebreathing mask.
- Investigate the chief complaint, obtain a SAMPLE history, and arrange for prompt transport to a medical facility.
- Let the responding crew know that standard precautions are being followed, including use of a HEPA respirator. This information will better prepare the crew to handle the patient. (page 28)

Skills

Skill Drills

Skill Drill 2-1: Proper Removal of Medical Gloves

1. Partially remove the first glove by pinching at the wrist. Be careful to touch only the outside of the glove.

2. Remove the second glove by pinching the exterior with the partially gloved hand.

3. Pull the second glove inside out toward the fingertips.

4. Grasp both gloves with your free hand, touching only the clean interior surfaces, and gently remove the gloves. (page 30)

Chapter 3: Medical, Legal, and Ethical Issues

General Knowledge

Matching

1. D (page 40)	**3.** F (page 42)	**5.** C (page 44)	**7.** I (page 42)	**9.** G (page 41)
2. B (page 40)	**4.** H (page 41)	**6.** J (page 39)	**8.** A (page 39)	**10.** E (page 42)

Multiple Choice

1. B (page 45)	**6.** C (page 40)	**11.** C (page 40)	**16.** A (page 41)	**21.** A (page 45)
2. C (page 40)	**7.** A (page 42)	**12.** A (page 40)	**17.** A (page 41)	**22.** D (page 44)
3. D (page 44)	**8.** C (page 42)	**13.** A (page 40)	**18.** B (page 41)	**23.** D (page 44)
4. A (page 42)	**9.** D (page 39)	**14.** B (page 40)	**19.** C (page 40)	**24.** C (pages 44–45)
5. D (page 39)	**10.** D (page 40)	**15.** D (page 40)	**20.** C (page 42)	**25.** B (page 45)

True/False

1. T (page 39)	**4.** T (page 45)	**7.** T (page 45)	**10.** F (page 40)	**13.** T (page 44)
2. F (page 40)	**5.** F (page 40)	**8.** F (page 46)	**11.** T (page 41)	**14.** T (page 45)
3. T (page 44)	**6.** T (page 40)	**9.** T (page 39)	**12.** F (page 42)	**15.** F (page 45)

Crossword Puzzle

Critical Thinking

Fill-in-the-Blank

1. living will (advance directive) (pages 41–42)
2. negligence (page 44)
3. good faith (page 45)
4. competent (page 41)
5. Expressed (page 40)
6. minor (page 40)
7. durable power of attorney (page 41)
8. HIPAA (page 44)
9. protected (page 45)
10. accurate; readable (page 46)

Short Answer

1. The United States Department of Transportation developed the educational standards for EMRs. (page 40)
2. The purpose of Good Samaritan laws is to protect citizens from liability for errors or omissions in giving good faith emergency care. (page 45)
3. 1. Decapitation
   2. Rigor mortis
   3. Tissue decomposition
   4. Dependent lividity (page 42)
4. Any three of the following:
   - Knife wounds
   - Gunshot wounds
   - Motor vehicle collisions
   - Suspected child abuse
   - Domestic violence
   - Elder abuse
   - Dog bites
   - Rape (page 45)
5. Any three of the following:
   - Condition of the patient when found
   - Patient's description of the injury or illness
   - Patient's initial and repeat vital signs
   - Treatment you gave
   - Agency and personnel who took over treatment of the patient
   - Any reportable conditions present
   - Any infectious disease exposure
   - Anything unusual regarding the case (page 46)

You Make the Call

1. Your answer should include the following steps and information:
   - Assess scene safety and take steps to protect yourself.
   - If the scene is unsafe, wait until law enforcement personnel give the signal that the scene is safe for entry.
   - Make patient care your first priority after personal safety.

- Document anything at the scene that seems unusual.
- Move the patient only if necessary, and take a mental snapshot of the scene before you do.
- Touch only what you need to touch to gain access to the patient.
- Preserve the crime scene for further investigation, and do not move anything unless it interferes with your ability to provide care.
- Be careful not to cut through knife or bullet holes in the patient's clothing.
- Be careful not to alter or destroy evidence when placing your equipment.
- Keep nonessential personnel, such as curious bystanders, away from the scene.
- Work with the appropriate law enforcement authorities on the scene to ensure that everyone has the information they need.
- After you have attended to the patient(s), write a short report about the incident, and make a sketch of the scene that shows how and where you found the patient. (page 45)

2. Your answer should include the following steps and information:

- Unless this patient shows indications of obvious death (eg, decapitation, rigor mortis, tissue decomposition, dependent lividity), you need to begin resuscitation and continue until someone of higher training assumes care or a physician provides you with an order to cease resuscitation.
- Even though the expressed wishes of this patient may be to have absolutely no resuscitation, because there is not a valid legal DNR order or advance directive available to confirm this, appropriate medical care must be initiated.
- Consult your local protocols and state regulations for specific DNR guidelines in your state. (pages 41–42)

Chapter 4: Communications and Documentation

General Knowledge

Matching

1. E (page 51) **3.** C (page 52) **5.** G (page 52) **7.** H (page 51)

2. B (page 52) **4.** D (page 52) **6.** A (page 52) **8.** F (page 52)

Multiple Choice

1. C (page 55) **5.** C (page 56) **9.** A (page 58) **13.** C (page 59) **17.** B (page 55)

2. B (page 54) **6.** C (page 57) **10.** A (page 51) **14.** D (page 61)

3. A (page 54) **7.** B (page 57) **11.** C (page 56) **15.** B (page 61)

4. D (page 55) **8.** B (page 58) **12.** B (pages 58–59) **16.** C (page 53)

True/False

1. T (page 55) **4.** F (pages 61, 63) **7.** F (page 59) **10.** T (page 59) **13.** T (page 53)

2. T (page 54) **5.** T (page 63) **8.** T (page 58) **11.** T (page 53)

3. F (page 51) **6.** T (page 60) **9.** F (page 60) **12.** F (page 54)

Crossword Puzzle

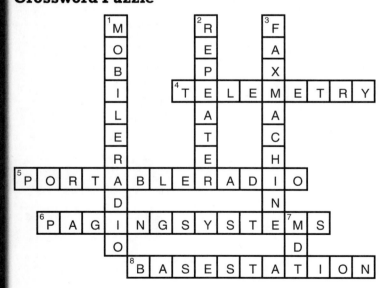

Critical Thinking

Fill-in-the-Blank

1. phone; radio (page 52)
2. mobile (page 51)
3. physical; mental (page 59)
4. Federal Communications Commission (page 51)
5. deaf (page 59)
6. professional (page 59)
7. Hypertension (page 61)
8. Documentation (page 61)
9. radio (page 52)
10. medical control (page 54)

Fill-in-the-Table (page 61)

Prefixes Commonly Used in Medical Terminology	
Prefix	**Meaning**
Brady-	**Slow**
Tachy-	**Rapid or swift**
Therm-	In relation to quantities of heat
Hyper-	Above, excessive, or beyond
Hypo-	**Below, underneath, or deficient**
Naso-	Denoting the nose
Oro-	**Denoting the mouth**
Arterio-	**Relationship to an artery**
Cardio-	Heart
Hem-, hema-, hemo-	**Blood**
Neuro-	Denoting nerve, nervous system, or nervous tissue
Vaso-	Vessel, as in blood vessel

Short Answer

1. A base station is a powerful, stationary two-way radio that is attached to one or more fixed antennas. A mobile radio is mounted in a vehicle and draws electricity from the electrical system of the vehicle. (page 51)
2. 1. Data
   2. Voice (page 51)
3. A portable radio is a two-way radio with a self-contained battery, a built-in microphone, and a built-in antenna. (page 52)
4. 1. Paging systems
   2. Mobile data terminals
   3. Fax machines (page 52)
5. Telemetry is used to transmit electrocardiograms and other patient data to online medical control. (page 52)
6. This gives the patient, family members, and bystanders an idea of who you are and lets them know your qualifications. (page 56)
7. Technical medical terms may frighten or confuse the patient. (page 56)

8. **1.** Assess the situation. Try to determine the cause of the patient's disruptive behavior.

2. Protect the patient and yourself.

3. Stay between the patient and an exit whenever possible.

4. Do not take your eyes off the patient or turn your back.

5. If the patient has a weapon, stay clear and wait for law enforcement personnel, no matter how badly injured the patient seems to be.

6. As soon as your personal safety is ensured, carry out the appropriate emergency medical care. (page 60)

You Make the Call

1. Your hand-off report should include the following information:

- The age and sex of the patient
- The history of the incident
- The patient's chief complaint
- The patient's level of responsiveness
- A description of how you found the patient
- The status of the vital signs, airway, breathing, and circulation (including severe bleeding)
- The results of the physical examination
- A report of any pertinent medical conditions with the SAMPLE format
- A report of the interventions provided (page 54)

2. Your answer should include the following steps and information:

- Identify yourself by showing the patient your patch or badge.
- Touch the patient; a deaf patient needs human contact just as much as a hearing patient.
- Face the patient when you speak so he can see your lips and facial expressions.
- Speak slowly and distinctly; do not shout.
- Watch the patient's face for expressions of understanding or uncertainty.
- Repeat or rephrase your comments in clear, simple language.
- If all of these attempts at communication fail, write down your questions, and offer a paper and pencil to allow the patient to respond. (page 58)

Chapter 5: The Human Body

General Knowledge

Matching

1. K (page 72)	**4.** I (page 72)	**7.** H (page 70)	**10.** J (page 70)	**13.** F (page 70)
2. B (page 72)	**5.** D (page 72)	**8.** L (page 70)	**11.** M (pages 72–73)	**14.** E (page 70)
3. G (page 72)	**6.** A (page 69)	**9.** O (page 70)	**12.** C (page 70)	**15.** N (page 69)

Multiple Choice

1. B (pages 75–76)	**9.** B (page 70)	**17.** B (page 73)	**25.** B (page 72)	**33.** D (page 70)
2. C (page 76)	**10.** C (page 76)	**18.** A (page 74)	**26.** B (page 72)	**34.** C (page 70)
3. D (page 71)	**11.** C (page 76)	**19.** D (page 73)	**27.** A (page 72)	**35.** D (page 70)
4. C (page 72)	**12.** D (page 75)	**20.** D (page 73)	**28.** C (page 72)	**36.** A (page 70)
5. C (page 73)	**13.** D (page 75)	**21.** B (page 72)	**29.** D (page 71)	**37.** C (page 70)
6. A (page 70)	**14.** B (page 75)	**22.** D (page 72)	**30.** A (page 69)	**38.** D (page 77)
7. B (pages 70–71)	**15.** B (page 75)	**23.** A (page 72)	**31.** B (page 69)	**39.** C (page 77)
8. C (page 70)	**16.** D (page 73)	**24.** B (page 72)	**32.** C (page 70)	**40.** C (page 79)

True/False

1. F (page 75)	**5.** T (page 72)	**9.** F (page 70)	**13.** T (page 72)	**17.** T (page 75)
2. T (page 75)	**6.** F (page 69)	**10.** T (page 70)	**14.** F (page 73)	**18.** T (page 76)
3. F (page 71)	**7.** T (page 69)	**11.** F (page 70)	**15.** F (page 75)	**19.** F (page 75)
4. F (page 71)	**8.** T (page 69)	**12.** F (pages 71–72)	**16.** F (page 75)	**20.** T (page 75)

Labeling

1. **The Respiratory System**
   - **A.** Upper airway
   - **B.** Trachea
   - **C.** Lung
   - **D.** Diaphragm
   - **E.** Ribs
   - **F.** Bronchi (page 70)
2. **The Airway**
   - **A.** Nasal cavity (nasopharynx)
   - **B.** Mouth (oropharynx)
   - **C.** Epiglottis
   - **D.** Larynx
   - **E.** Esophagus
   - **F.** Trachea (windpipe)
   - **G.** Lung (page 70)
3. **The Circulatory System**
   - **A.** Lungs
   - **B.** Heart
   - **C.** Aorta (artery)
   - **D.** Inferior vena cava (major vein) (page 71)
4. **The Rib Cage**
   - **A.** Sternum (breastbone)
   - **B.** Ribs
   - **C.** Cartilage
   - **D.** Xiphoid process
   - **E.** Floating ribs (page 74)
5. **The Digestive System**
   - **A.** Mouth
   - **B.** Pharynx (throat)
   - **C.** Esophagus
   - **D.** Liver
   - **E.** Stomach
   - **F.** Gallbladder
   - **G.** Pancreas
   - **H.** Large intestine
   - **I.** Small intestine
   - **J.** Rectum
   - **K.** Anus (page 76)

Crossword Puzzle

Across:
1. SHOULDER GIRDLES
4. STERNUM
6. CARTILAGE
7. NERVOUS SYSTEM
8. TENDONS
10. FLOATING RIBS
11. JOINT
12. VERTEBRAE

Down:
2. HUMERUS
3. GENITO (GENIT...ION)
5. PLASMA
9. INSULIN

Critical Thinking

Fill-in-the-Blank

1. Twelve (page 73)
2. vertebrae (page 72)
3. spinal cord (page 72)
4. jawbone (page 72)
5. floating (page 73)
6. fibula (page 74)
7. joint (page 74)
8. heart (page 75)
9. abdomen (page 75)
10. mouth (page 75)

Fill-in-the-Table (page 79)

Typical Vital Sign Values Based on Age			
Age	Pulse (Heart Rate)(beats/min)	Respirations (breaths/min)	Blood Pressure (mm Hg)
Infants (newborn to age 1 year)	100-160	**25-50**	50-95 systolic
Children (ages 1 to **8** years)	**70-150**	15-30	80-110 systolic
Adults	60-100	12-20	**90-140** systolic

Short Answer

1. Nasal cavity (nasopharynx); mouth (oropharynx); larynx (voice box); trachea (windpipe); lung (page 70)
2. Protect against harmful substances in the environment; regulate body temperature; transmit information from the outside environment to the brain (page 76)
3. Support the body; protect vital structures; manufacture red blood cells (page 72)
4. Contracting (shortening); relaxing (lengthening) (page 75)
5. Cervical spine (neck); thoracic spine (upper back); lumbar spine (lower back); sacrum (base of spine); coccyx (tailbone) (page 72)
6. Mouth; throat; esophagus; stomach; small intestine; large intestine; rectum; anus (page 75)
7. Skull; spine; shoulder girdles; upper extremity; rib cage; pelvis; lower extremity (pages 72–74)

You Make the Call

1. Your answer should include the following steps and information:
   - Check the pulse at the carotid artery at either side of the neck.
   - Check the radial artery at the wrist.
   - Check the femoral artery on the inside of the upper leg. (page 71)
2. Your answer should include the following information:
   - The skin protects against harmful substances in the environment, including foreign substances, bacteria, and viruses. This patient is at risk of infection if his burns go untreated.
   - The skin regulates body temperature. When the body temperature is too high, small blood vessels in the skin dilate and bring more blood to the surface of the skin, where the heat is transferred to the air. Because this patient has potentially lost skin from burns, he will not be able to maintain adequate body temperature.
   - Skin transmits information from the outside environment to the brain. Skin receives information from the environment such as touch, pressure, and pain. It also senses heat and cold. This patient is transmitting sensations of pain and heat to the brain as a result of the burned skin. He will continue to experience these unpleasant feelings until he is able to receive definitive care at a tertiary facility such as a burn center. (pages 76–77)

Chapter 6: Airway Management

General Knowledge

Matching

1. D (page 91)	**4.** A (page 91)	**7.** I (page 91)	**10.** M (page 121)	**13.** N (page 92)
2. G (page 91)	**5.** K (pages 95–96)	**8.** F (page 118)	**11.** H (page 120)	**14.** L (page 103)
3. E (page 92)	**6.** B (page 99)	**9.** C (page 92)	**12.** O (page 91)	**15.** J (pages 90–91)

Multiple Choice

1. A (page 93)	**9.** B (page 92)	**17.** B (page 103)	**25.** D (pages 91–92)	**33.** B (page 99)
2. D (page 93)	**10.** A (page 103)	**18.** C (page 112)	**26.** B (page 92)	**34.** B (pages 103, 110)
3. D (page 95)	**11.** D (page 103)	**19.** C (pages 112–113)	**27.** C (page 93)	**35.** D (page 103)
4. C (page 96)	**12.** C (page 103)	**20.** B (page 113)	**28.** D (page 95)	**36.** A (pages 104–105)
5. A (page 97)	**13.** A (page 103)	**21.** A (page 119)	**29.** C (page 97)	**37.** B (pages 120–121)
6. B (page 100)	**14.** D (page 110)	**22.** A (page 119)	**30.** A (page 102)	**38.** A (page 121)
7. C (page 100)	**15.** B (page 110)	**23.** A (page 91)	**31.** C (pages 102–103)	
8. B (page 93)	**16.** A (pages 110, 122)	**24.** B (page 91)	**32.** D (page 97)	

True/False

1. T (page 91)	**8.** T (page 121)	**15.** T (page 102)	**22.** F (page 93)	**29.** F (page 110)
2. T (page 112)	**9.** F (page 121)	**16.** F (page 103)	**23.** T (page 97)	**30.** T (page 111)
3. F (page 113)	**10.** T (page 121)	**17.** T (page 97)	**24.** T (pages 99–100)	**31.** T (page 112)
4. F (page 111)	**11.** F (page 95)	**18.** T (page 91)	**25.** F (pages 99–100)	**32.** F (page 119)
5. T (page 112)	**12.** T (page 95)	**19.** F (page 92)	**26.** T (page 102)	**33.** F (page 121)
6. T (page 112)	**13.** T (page 97)	**20.** F (page 111)	**27.** T (page 105)	**34.** T (page 107)
7. T (pages 112–113)	**14.** T (page 100)	**21.** T (page 93)	**28.** F (page 110)	**35.** F (page 107)

Labeling

1. Airway Maintenance
   A. Oral airways (page 99)
   B. Battery-powered suction device (page 96)
   C. Nasal airways (page 100)

2. Assisted Ventilation
   A. Barrier devices (page 105)
   B. Bag-mask device (page 106)

Crossword Puzzle

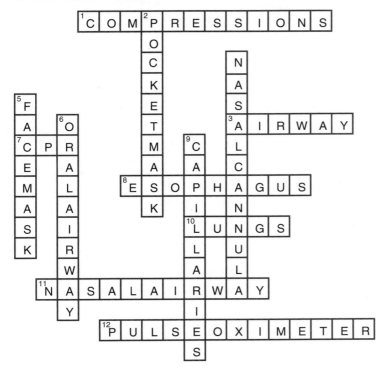

Critical Thinking

Fill-in-the-Blank

1. manual; mechanical (page 95)
2. recovery (page 97)
3. cyanosis (or blue skin) (page 99)
4. respiratory arrest (page 102)
5. nose (page 103)

6. carbon dioxide (page 92)
7. 4; 6 (page 91)
8. nasal (page 101)
9. check; correct (page 90)
10. earlobe; mouth (page 99)

Short Answer

1. Maintain airway; maintain pathway for suction (page 99)
2. 1. Select the proper size.
    2. Open the mouth with one hand after manually opening the patient's airway with a head tilt–chin lift or jaw-thrust maneuver.
    3. Hold the oral airway upside down with the other hand. Insert the airway gently along the roof of the mouth until it meets resistance.
    4. Rotate the airway 180 degrees until the flange comes to rest on the patient's teeth or lips. (page 99)
3. 1. Select the proper size.
    2. Coat the airway with a water-soluble lubricant.
    3. Select the larger nostril.
    4. Gently stretch the nostril open with your thumb.
    5. Gently insert the airway until the flange rests against the nose. (pages 101–102)

4. **1.** Position yourself at the patient's head.

2. Open the patient's airway.

3. Place the mask over the mouth and nose of the patient.

4. Grasp the mask and the patient's jaw.

5. Maintain an airtight seal.

6. Take a deep breath and seal your mouth over the mouthpiece.

7. Breathe slowly into the patient for 1 second, breathing until the patient's chest rises.

8. Monitor the patient for proper head position, air exchange, and vomiting. (pages 104–105)

5. Any two of the following:

- Noisy respirations (including wheezing or gurgling)
- Rapid or gasping respirations
- Cyanosis (blue skin)
- Lack of chest movements
- Lack of breath sounds
- Lack of air against the side of your face (page 102)

6. Mild (partial); severe (complete) (page 112)

7. Roll the patient as a unit to the side, supporting the head, and place the patient's face on its side so that secretions can run out of the mouth. (pages 97, 99)

8. You do not have to enter the automobile.

You can easily monitor the patient's carotid pulse and breathing patterns by using your fingers.

It stabilizes the patient's cervical spine.

It opens the patient's airway. (page 124)

You Make the Call

1. Your answer should include the following steps and information:

- Ask "Are you choking? Can you speak?"
- Stand behind the patient.
- Position your hands for abdominal thrusts.
- Repeat abdominal thrusts until the object is expelled or the patient becomes unconscious. (pages 114–115)

2. Your answer should include the following steps and information:

- Keep the patient's neck straight; do not hyperextend the patient's head and neck.
- Examine the stoma, and clean any mucus present in it.
- If there is a breathing tube in the opening, remove it to make sure the tube is clear. Clean the tube rapidly and replace it in the stoma.
- Place your bag-mask device over the stoma and begin to ventilate.
- Watch for chest rise. If the chest does not rise, the patient may be a partial neck breather. If this is the case, you will need to seal the mouth and nose when ventilating the stoma. (page 121)

Skills

Skill Drills

Skill Drill 6-2: Inserting an Oral Airway

1. Size the airway by measuring from the patient's **earlobe** to the corner of the mouth.

2. Insert the **oral airway** upside down along the roof of the patient's mouth until you feel resistance.

3. Rotate the airway **180** degrees until the flange comes to rest on the patient's lips or teeth. (page 100)

Skill Drill 6-3: Inserting a Nasal Airway

  1. Size the **airway** by measuring from the tip of the patient's nose to the patient's earlobe.
  2. Insert the lubricated airway into the **larger** nostril.
  3. Advance the airway until the flange rests against the **nose**. (page 101)

Skill Drill 6-6: Using a Bag-Mask Device With One Rescuer

  1. Kneel at the patient's **head** and maintain an open airway. Check the patient's mouth for **fluids**, foreign bodies, and **dentures**.
  2. Select the proper **mask** size.
  3. Place the mask over the patient's **face**.
  4. **Seal** the mask.
  5. **Squeeze** the bag with your other hand. Check for chest **rise**.
  6. Add **supplemental oxygen**. (page 108)

Skill Drill 6-7: Performing Infant Rescue Breathing

  1. Establish the patient's level of **responsiveness**.
  2. Open the infant's airway using the **head tilt-chin lift** maneuver.
  3. Check for **breathing**.
  4. Perform infant **rescue** breathing. (page 113)

Chapter 7: Professional Rescuer CPR

General Knowledge

Matching

1. F (page 132)	**3.** G (page 132)	**5.** A (page 139)	**7.** E (page 132)	**9.** I (page 148)
2. D (page 137)	**4.** H (page 132)	**6.** C (page 132)	**8.** J (page 137)	**10.** B (page 132)

Multiple Choice

1. A (page 134)	**8.** C (page 139)	**15.** A (page 143)	**22.** D (page 135)	**29.** B (page 153)
2. D (page 132)	**9.** B (page 139)	**16.** C (page 148)	**23.** D (pages 135, 156)	**30.** C (page 131)
3. C (page 135)	**10.** B (page 144)	**17.** B (page 139)	**24.** B (page 133)	
4. B (page 137)	**11.** D (page 145)	**18.** D (page 131)	**25.** C (page 134)	
5. D (page 137)	**12.** D (page 145)	**19.** C (page 132)	**26.** A (page 148)	
6. D (page 139)	**13.** D (page 146)	**20.** A (page 139)	**27.** C (page 149)	
7. D (page 141)	**14.** D (pages 145, 148)	**21.** C (page 150)	**28.** D (pages 132–133)	

True/False

1. T (page 134)	**8.** T (page 133)	**15.** F (page 139)	**22.** F (page 135)	**29.** T (page 146)
2. T (page 136)	**9.** T (page 131)	**16.** F (page 141)	**23.** T (page 135)	**30.** T (page 135)
3. T (page 136)	**10.** T (page 136)	**17.** T (page 139)	**24.** T (page 135)	**31.** T (page 151)
4. F (page 136)	**11.** F (page 134)	**18.** F (page 141)	**25.** F (page 136)	**32.** T (page 152)
5. T (page 149)	**12.** T (page 133)	**19.** F (page 149)	**26.** T (page 145)	
6. F (page 149)	**13.** F (page 139)	**20.** T (page 149)	**27.** F (page 144)	
7. T (page 149)	**14.** T (page 139)	**21.** F (page 152)	**28.** F (page 148)	

Labeling

1. Pulse Locations
   A. Neck; carotid pulse
   B. Wrist; radial pulse
   C. Arm; brachial pulse
   D. Groin; femoral pulse (page 132)

Crossword Puzzle

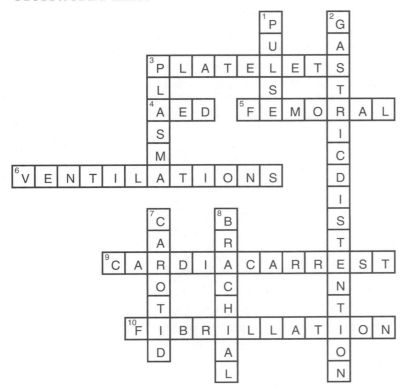

Critical Thinking

Fill-in-the-Blank

1. 100 (page 145)
2. brachial (page 144)
3. pump (heart); fluid (blood) (page 131)
4. aorta (page 132)
5. Rigor mortis (page 134)
6. gastric distention (page 148)

7. ventricular fibrillation (page 149)
8. standard precautions (page 135)
9. 4; 6 (page 133)
10. recertification (page 152)

Short Answer

1. Maintain the head tilt (page 137)
2. Just below the nipple line over the sternum (page 137)
3. Too much air delivered too fast; partial obstruction of the airway (page 148)
4. Neck or carotid artery, groin or femoral artery, wrist or radial artery, and arm or brachial artery (page 132)
5. Decapitation, rigor mortis, evidence of tissue decomposition, and dependent lividity (pages 134–135)
6. • If the patient is wet, dry the patient before initiating defibrillation.
   • If the patient has a pacemaker, you may need to reposition one of the defibrillator pads so it is not directly over the pacemaker.
   • If the patient has a transdermal medication patch on his or her chest, remove the patch and wipe the skin before defibrillating the patient. (page 152)

7. 1. Effective spontaneous circulation and ventilation are restored.

   2. Resuscitation efforts are transferred to another trained person who continues CPR.

   3. A physician orders you to stop.

   4. The patient is transferred to properly trained EMS personnel.

   5. Reliable criteria for death are recognized.

   6. You are too exhausted to continue resuscitation, environmental hazards endanger your safety, or continued resuscitation would place the lives of others at risk. (page 135)

8. 1. A second rescuer feels a carotid pulse while you are compressing the chest.

   2. The patient's skin color improves (from blue to pink).

   3. The chest visibly rises during ventilations.

   4. Compressions and ventilations are delivered at the appropriate rate and depth. (page 148)

You Make the Call

1. Your answer should include the following steps and information:
   - Introduce yourself.
   - Check responsiveness (if unresponsive, check for breathing and a pulse, and start CPR if needed).
   - Check and correct the airway (including the use of proper techniques for opening the airway).
   - Check and correct breathing (including the use of proper method of performing rescue breathing).
   - Check and correct circulation (including correct steps of external cardiac compressions).
   - Establish the need for additional resources.
   - Establish the need to arrange immediate transportation. (pages 137–139)

2. Your answer should include the following steps and information:
   - This woman is exhibiting the reliable sign of death called dependent lividity.
   - The history given by the neighbor and the presentation of the patient clearly indicate that the woman has been dead for anywhere from several hours to several days; therefore, CPR should not be initiated for this patient.
   - In this situation, contact your local law enforcement agency (if not already present), and follow your local protocols for dealing with deceased patients. (pages 134–135)

Skills

Skill Drills

Skill Drill 7-1: Performing Adult Chest Compressions

1. Locate the **top** and **bottom** of the sternum. Place the **heel** of your hand in the center of the chest, in between the nipples.

2. Place your other hand on top of your first hand and **interlock** your fingers.

3. Compress the chest of an adult **at least 2"** straight down. (page 136)

Skill Drill 7-2: Performing One-Rescuer Adult CPR

1. Establish responsiveness and lack of breathing.

2. Check for circulation.

3. Perform chest compressions. (page 138)

4. Open the airway.

5. Perform rescue breathing.

Skill Drill 7-5: Procedure for Automated External Defibrillation

1. Check for **responsiveness**, **breathing**, and circulation.

2. If the patient is unresponsive, not breathing, and **pulseless**, begin providing chest compressions.

3. Apply the **adhesive pads** and connect them to the defibrillator. Turn on the AED. Do not touch the **patient**. Allow the AED to **analyze** the rhythm.

4. Determine whether a **shock** is advised by the defibrillator. If a shock is advised, defibrillate the patient.

5. As soon as the AED gives the shock, perform **five** cycles of CPR (about 2 minutes), starting with **chest compressions**, then analyze the rhythm. If the AED advises no shock, perform five cycles of CPR (about 2 minutes), starting with chest compressions, then **analyze** the rhythm. (pages 150–151)

Chapter 8: Patient Assessment

General Knowledge

Matching

1. F (page 176)	**3.** G (page 181)	**5.** D (page 182)	**7.** J (page 175)	**9.** I (page 168)
2. C (page 182)	**4.** A (page 172)	**6.** H (page 175)	**8.** B (page 181)	**10.** E (page 175)

Multiple Choice

1. D (page 164)	**9.** C (page 175)	**17.** A (page 181)	**25.** A (page 170)	**33.** C (page 184)
2. C (page 168)	**10.** C (page 179)	**18.** C (page 170)	**26.** D (page 170)	**34.** D (page 180)
3. C (page 170)	**11.** D (page 168)	**19.** D (page 164)	**27.** B (page 180)	**35.** C (page 176)
4. A (page 169)	**12.** D (page 168)	**20.** B (page 165)	**28.** D (page 180)	**36.** B (pages 178–179)
5. A (page 180)	**13.** B (page 168)	**21.** A (page 165)	**29.** C (pages 181–182)	**37.** B (page 179)
6. D (page 181)	**14.** D (page 169)	**22.** D (page 170)	**30.** C (page 183)	**38.** C (page 170)
7. B (page 181)	**15.** A (page 181)	**23.** C (page 170)	**31.** A (page 183)	**39.** A (page 172)
8. C (page 181)	**16.** D (page 181)	**24.** B (page 170)	**32.** D (page 184)	**40.** B (page 175)

True/False

1. T (page 164)	**9.** T (page 169)	**17.** T (page 168)	**25.** T (page 172)	**33.** F (page 181)
2. T (page 166)	**10.** F (pages 169–170)	**18.** T (page 169)	**26.** F (page 164)	**34.** F (page 181)
3. T (page 164)	**11.** F (page 172)	**19.** F (page 168)	**27.** F (page 175)	**35.** T (page 181)
4. F (page 164)	**12.** T (page 175)	**20.** T (page 169)	**28.** T (page 175)	**36.** F (page 183)
5. T (page 165)	**13.** F (page 172)	**21.** F (page 169)	**29.** T (page 175)	**37.** F (page 176)
6. F (page 165)	**14.** T (page 168)	**22.** T (page 169)	**30.** T (page 180)	**38.** F (pages 178–179)
7. T (page 168)	**15.** F (page 170)	**23.** T (page 170)	**31.** T (page 180)	**39.** T (page 179)
8. F (page 168)	**16.** F (page 168)	**24.** T (page 169)	**32.** T (page 180)	**40.** T (page 180)

Labeling

1. Pupil Size
   A. Normal pupil
   B. Dilated pupil
   C. Constricted pupil (page 183)

Crossword Puzzle

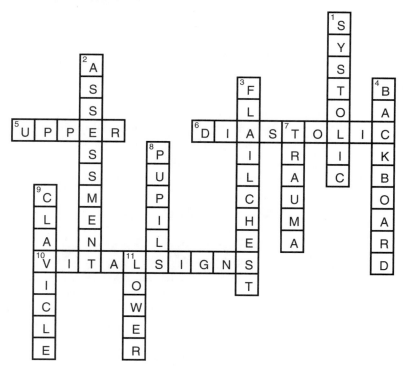

Critical Thinking

Fill-in-the-Blank

1. introduce yourself (page 168)
2. unresponsive (page 168)
3. head tilt–chin lift (page 169)
4. rate; quality (page 169)
5. airway (page 169)
6. symptom (page 175)
7. sign (page 175)
8. serious illness (page 181)
9. shock (page 181)
10. rate; rhythm; quality (page 181)

11. 98.6°F (37°C) (page 183)
12. respiration; pulse; blood pressure; skin condition (page 175)
13. **A.** 4
    B. 2
    C. 1
    D. 5
    E. 3
    F. 6 (pages 168–170)
14. Hypertension (page 182)

15. brachial (page 182)
16. palpation (page 182)
17. primary (page 186)
18. medial (page 180)
19. head-to-toe (page 175)
20. standard precautions (page 166)

Fill-in-the-Table (page 176)

Skin Color		
Color	**Term**	**Sign of:**
Red	Flushed	Fever or sunburn
White	Pale	Shock
Blue	Cyanotic	Airway obstruction
Yellow	Jaundiced	Liver disease

Short Answer

1. 1. Scene size-up
    2. Primary assessment
    3. History taking
    4. Secondary assessment
    5. Reassessment (page 162)

2. Any three of the following:
    - Location of incident
    - Main problem or type of incident
    - Number of people involved
    - Safety level of the scene (page 164)

3. 1. Review dispatch information
    2. Ensure scene safety
    3. Determine the mechanism of injury or nature of illness
    4. Take standard precautions
    5. Determine the number of patients
    6. Consider additional resources (pages 164–166)

4. Any four of the following:
    - Motor vehicle crash
    - Fallen electrical wires
    - Traffic
    - Spilled gasoline
    - Unstable building
    - Crime scene
    - Crowds
    - Unstable surfaces (eg, slopes, ice, and water)
    - Electricity
    - Hazardous materials
    - Poisonous fumes
    - Water
    - Weather
    - Biological hazards (page 164)

5. How the accident happened; type of accident; extent of damage (page 165)

6. Alert; verbal; pain; unresponsive (pages 168–169)

7. Place the side of your face by the patient's nose and mouth and check for signs of breathing. (page 169)

8. Deformity; open injuries; tenderness; swelling (page 175)

9. 1. Radial artery, found on the wrist; used for responsive adult patients
    2. Carotid artery, found on the sides of the neck; used for unresponsive adult patients
    3. Brachial artery, found on the arm; used for infants (page 181)

10. Squeeze the patient's nail bed firmly between your thumb and forefinger, then release the pressure. Determine the length of time it takes for the nail bed to become pink again. (page 181)

11. Signs and symptoms; allergies; medications; pertinent past medical history; last oral intake; events leading up to this illness or injury (pages 172–173)

12. Head; eyes; nose; mouth; neck; face; chest; abdomen; pelvis; back; extremities (pages 175–179)

13. Fingernail beds; whites of eyes; palms of the hands; inside of mouth (page 170)

14. 1. Provide the age and sex of the patient.
    2. Describe the history of the incident.
    3. Describe the patient's primary or chief complaint.
    4. Describe the patient's level of responsiveness.
    5. Report the status of the vital signs: airway, breathing, and circulation (including severe bleeding).
    6. Describe the results of the secondary patient assessment.
    7. Report any pertinent medical conditions using the SAMPLE format.
    8. Report the interventions provided. (page 186)

You Make the Call

1. Your answer should include the following steps and information:
   - Perform a thorough scene size-up, including ensuring scene safety, taking standard precautions, and obtaining additional help.
   - Introduce yourself to the patient and family, and attempt to assess the level of responsiveness.
   - Assess and correct, if necessary, airway, breathing, and circulation.
   - Provide an update to the responding EMS unit.
   - Attempt to gather as much SAMPLE history as possible.
   - Perform a secondary assessment, including a head-to-toe physical examination.
   - Obtain a set of vital signs, including pulse, respiration, capillary refill, blood pressure, pupil size and reactivity, level of responsiveness, and skin condition.
   - Provide a hand-off verbal report to the EMS unit upon their arrival. (pages 164–186)

2. Your answer should include the following steps and information:
   - Wrap the blood pressure cuff around the upper arm, making sure the bottom of the cuff is 1″ to 2″ above the crease of the elbow, and the arrow is pointing to the brachial artery.
   - Make sure the valve of the cuff is closed in one hand, and assess the radial pulse with the other hand.
   - Place the earpieces of the stethoscope in your ears and the diaphragm over the brachial artery.
   - Slowly pump up the blood pressure cuff until you can no longer feel the radial pulse.
   - Continue to pump for an additional 30 mm Hg beyond the disappearance of the radial pulse.
   - Slowly and smoothly release air from the cuff by opening the control valve at a rate of 2 to 4 mm per second.
   - Carefully watch the needle indicator, listen for the pulse to return, and note the pressure reading when you first hear the pulse (systolic pressure).
   - As the cuff pressure continues to fall, listen for the moment when the pulse disappears (diastolic pressure).
   - Release the remainder of the air after determining the diastolic pressure by completely opening the cuff valve. (pages 182–183)

Chapter 9: Medical Emergencies

General Knowledge

Matching

1. H (page 207) **3.** G (page 204) **5.** E (page 209) **7.** I (page 207) **9.** C (page 204)
2. B (page 204) **4.** F (page 204) **6.** D (page 204) **8.** J (page 199) **10.** A (page 201)

Multiple Choice

1. A (page 209) **10.** A (page 204) **19.** D (page 208) **28.** B (page 209) **37.** D (pages 201–202)
2. C (page 201) **11.** C (page 204) **20.** D (page 209) **29.** A (page 209) **38.** A (pages 203–204)
3. D (page 203) **12.** C (page 205) **21.** C (page 209) **30.** B (pages 207–208) **39.** C (page 203)
4. B (page 201) **13.** C (page 205) **22.** B (page 209) **31.** C (pages 204–205) **40.** A (pages 203–204)
5. D (page 202) **14.** A (page 205) **23.** D (page 209) **32.** A (page 205) **41.** D (page 207)
6. C (page 201) **15.** C (page 205) **24.** C (pages 197–198) **33.** D (page 201) **42.** C (page 207)
7. A (page 202) **16.** D (pages 205, 207) **25.** D (page 199) **34.** D (page 201) **43.** A (pages 205, 207)
8. D (page 202) **17.** B (page 207) **26.** B (page 197) **35.** B (page 201) **44.** D (page 207)
9. A (pages 201–202) **18.** A (page 207) **27.** B (page 199) **36.** D (page 201) **45.** D (pages 207–208)

True/False

1. T (page 197) **7.** T (page 199) **13.** F (page 205) **19.** T (page 209) **25.** F (page 200)
2. F (page 198) **8.** F (page 198) **14.** F (page 204) **20.** F (page 198) **26.** T (page 214)
3. F (page 199) **9.** T (page 199) **15.** T (page 205) **21.** F (page 199) **27.** T (page 201)
4. T (page 200) **10.** T (page 207) **16.** F (page 205) **22.** F (page 199) **28.** T (page 204)
5. T (page 199) **11.** T (page 208) **17.** T (page 205) **23.** T (page 198) **29.** F (page 204)
6. F (page 199) **12.** T (page 205) **18.** T (page 205) **24.** F (page 198) **30.** T (page 204)

Crossword Puzzle

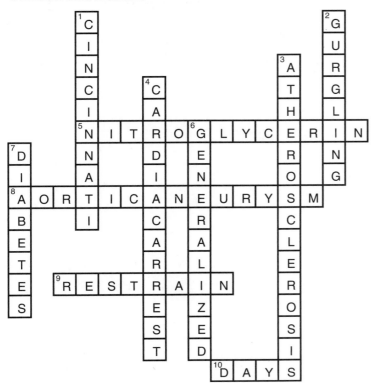

Critical Thinking

Fill-in-the-Blank

1. mental (page 198)
2. atherosclerosis (pages 200–201)
3. Seizures (page 198)
4. asthma attack (page 204)
5. 30; 45 (page 200)

6. AVPU (page 198)
7. emphysema (page 204)
8. Strokes (page 204)
9. shunt (page 209)
10. acute abdomen (page 209)

Fill-in-the-Table (page 208)

Comparing Insulin Shock and Diabetic Coma	
Insulin Shock	**Diabetic Coma**
Pale, moist, cool skin	**Warm, dry** skin
Rapid, weak pulse	**Rapid** pulse
Normal breathing	**Deep, rapid** breathing
Dizziness or headache	–
Confusion or unconsciousness	**Unresponsiveness** or unconsciousness
Rapid onset of symptoms (**minutes**)	**Slow** onset of symptoms (**days**)

Short Answer

1. Diabetic coma; insulin shock (pages 205, 207–208)
2. "Are you a diabetic?," "Did you take your insulin today?," "Have you eaten today?" (page 207)
3. Cola, orange juice, or honey (page 207)
4. Initial level of consciousness; any change in the patient's level of consciousness (page 198)
5. Any four of the following:
   - Head injury
   - Shock
   - Decreased level of oxygen to the brain
   - Stroke
   - Slow heart rate
   - High fever
   - Infection
   - Poisoning, including drugs and alcohol
   - Low level of blood glucose (diabetic emergencies)
   - Psychiatric condition
   - Insulin reaction (page 198)
6. Any five of the following:
   - Shortness of breath
   - Rapid, shallow breathing
   - Moist or gurgling respirations
   - Profuse sweating
   - Enlarged neck veins
   - Swollen ankles
   - Anxiety (page 203)
7. Facial droop, arm drift, and abnormal speech (page 205)

You Make the Call

1. Your answer should include the following steps and information:
   - This patient is showing signs and symptoms of insulin shock.
   - Summon for additional help or resources.
   - Perform a thorough physical examination.
   - Maintain ABCs.
   - Provide oxygen therapy.
   - Keep her warm.
   - Place her in the recovery position.
   - Do not give the patient anything to eat or drink due to her level of consciousness.
   - Prepare for prompt transportation. (pages 207–208)
2. Your answer should include the following steps and information:
   - This patient is showing signs and symptoms of congestive heart failure.
   - Place the patient in a sitting position and let his legs hang down.
   - Administer oxygen therapy in large quantities using a nonrebreathing mask.
   - Summon for additional help, and prepare the patient for prompt transport.
   - If the patient becomes unresponsive or goes into cardiac arrest, be prepared to perform the steps of CPR, if necessary. (pages 203–204)

Chapter 10: Poisoning and Substance Abuse

General Knowledge

Matching

1. G (page 220)
2. F (page 227)
3. I (page 227)
4. J (page 227)
5. C (page 227)
6. A (page 220)
7. E (page 227)
8. H (page 222)
9. D (page 219)
10. B (page 223)

Multiple Choice

1. B (page 218)
2. B (page 220)
3. C (page 219)
4. B (page 221)
5. D (page 224)
6. B (page 224)
7. B (page 227)
8. C (page 222)
9. B (page 217)
10. A (page 217)
11. D (page 217)
12. C (page 217)
13. D (page 219)
14. D (page 218)
15. A (page 219)
16. B (page 223)
17. B (page 221)
18. D (pages 220–221)
19. D (page 224)
20. C (page 222)
21. C (page 227)
22. D (page 224)
23. C (page 226)
24. B (page 227)
25. D (page 267)

True/False

1. F (page 218)
2. T (page 227)
3. T (page 219)
4. F (page 218)
5. F (page 219)
6. T (page 217)
7. F (page 218)
8. T (page 226)
9. F (page 222)
10. F (page 219)
11. T (page 218)
12. F (page 219)
13. F (page 219)
14. F (page 220)
15. F (page 220)
16. F (pages 220–221)
17. F (page 219)
18. T (page 222)
19. F (page 222)
20. T (page 222)
21. F (page 223)
22. T (page 223)
23. T (page 223)
24. T (pages 218, 224)
25. T (pages 223–224)
26. F (page 224)
27. T (page 224)
28. F (page 226)
29. F (page 226)
30. F (page 226)
31. T (page 227)

Crossword Puzzle

```
¹S  C  B  ²A
         N
         A        ³D
         P        E        ⁴B
         H        L        A
      ⁵D  R  Y  C  H  E  M  I  C  A  L  S
         L        R        E
      ⁶A  M  M  O  N  I  A
         C        U
         T        M
      ⁷I  N  G  E  S  T  I  O  N
         C        R        ⁸P
         S        E        O
         H     ⁹M  A  R  K  I  K  I  T
         O        E        S
     ¹⁰C  A  R  B  O  N  M  O  N  O  X  I  D  E
         K        S        N
```

Critical Thinking

Fill-in-the-Blank

1. **A.** ingested (page 218)
   B. inhaled (page 220)
   C. inhaled (page 220)
   D. injected (page 222)
   E. ingested (page 218)
   F. inhaled (page 220)
   G. absorbed (page 223)
2. ammonia; chlorine (page 227)
3. **A.** H
   B. A

C. B
D. B
E. H
F. A
G. H (page 267)
4. inhalants (page 227)
5. suicide (page 228)

Fill-in-the-Table (page 224)

Symptoms of Exposure to an Organophosphate Insecticide or Nerve Agent	
S	Salivation, sweating
L	Lacrimation (excessive tearing)
U	Urination
D	Defecation, diarrhea
G	Gastric upset
E	Emesis (vomiting)

Short Answer

1. Ingestion (page 218)
2. It will produce vomiting. (page 219)
3. Any five of the following:
   - Respiratory distress
   - Cough
   - Dizziness
   - Headache
   - Hoarseness
   - Chest pain
   - Confusion
   - Any other general signs and symptoms of poisoning (page 221)
4. Remove everyone from the dwelling, suspect carbon monoxide poisoning, and administer oxygen if available. (page 221)
5. It requires the use of a proper encapsulating suit with an SCBA. (page 220)
6. Any three of the following:
   - Itching
   - Hives
   - Swelling
   - Wheezing and severe respiratory distress
   - Generalized weakness
   - Unconsciousness
   - Rapid, weak pulse
   - Rapid, shallow breathing
   - Drop in blood pressure
   - Hypovolemic shock leading to cardiac arrest (pages 222–223)
7. Any four of the following:
   - Shock
   - Dizziness
   - Itching
   - Burning
   - Rash
   - Inflammation or redness of the skin
   - Nausea and vomiting
   - Traces of powder or liquid on the skin
   - Chemical burns
   - Any other general signs and symptoms of poisoning (page 224)

8. Provide basic life support, keep the patient from hurting himself or herself and others, provide reassurance and psychological support, and arrange for prompt transport to a medical facility. (page 228)

9. This should be done before any contact with water is made. (page 224)

You Make the Call

1. Your answer should include the following steps and information:
   - Assessment and maintenance of ABCs
   - Identification of the poison or type of medication that was taken
   - Contact with local poison control for direction of necessary care
   - Following directions from poison control
   - Arrangement of transport to an appropriate medical facility (page 218)

2. Your answer should include the following steps and information:
   - An active alarm in the home without signs of a fire and several people complaining of a headache should give you a high index of suspicion for carbon monoxide. In this case, make sure that everyone is removed from the residence and into fresh air.
   - Do not attempt to enter the house to search for others without protective equipment, such as SCBA, and enter only if you are trained.
   - It is important to remember that carbon monoxide is a colorless, odorless gas. Provide high-flow oxygen to those exposed to the gas and arrange for prompt transport to a medical facility. (pages 220–221)

Chapter 11: Behavioral Emergencies

General Knowledge

Matching

1. B (page 239)
2. D (page 236)
3. F (page 236)
4. H (page 246)
5. I (page 236)
6. J (page 244)
7. G (page 239)
8. E (page 244)
9. C (page 239)
10. A (page 236)

Multiple Choice

1. C (pages 236–237)
2. C (page 237)
3. D (page 239)
4. A (page 242)
5. D (pages 240, 242)
6. B (page 236)
7. D (page 236)
8. A (pages 236–237)
9. D (page 236)
10. C (page 236)
11. C (page 239)
12. B (page 239)
13. A (page 239)
14. B (page 242)
15. C (page 243)
16. D (page 244)
17. B (page 246)
18. A (page 245)
19. D (page 244)
20. A (page 243)

True/False

1. T (page 235)
2. T (page 236)
3. T (page 236)
4. F (page 236)
5. T (page 239)
6. T (page 239)
7. F (page 238)
8. T (page 239)
9. T (page 239)
10. T (pages 238–240)
11. F (page 239)
12. T (page 242)
13. T (page 236)
14. T (page 236)
15. T (page 236)
16. F (page 236)
17. F (page 236)
18. F (page 237)
19. F (page 237)
20. T (page 237)
21. F (page 235)
22. F (page 238)
23. T (pages 238–239)
24. F (page 239)
25. T (page 239)
26. T (page 239)
27. T (page 238)
28. F (page 239)
29. F (page 239)
30. T (page 239)
31. T (page 239)
32. T (page 239)
33. T (page 240)
34. T (page 240)
35. T (page 240)
36. T (page 240)
37. T (page 239)
38. F (page 242)
39. T (page 242)
40. T (page 243)
41. T (page 243)
42. F (page 244)
43. T (page 244)
44. F (page 245)
45. T (page 245)
46. T (pages 245–246)
47. T (page 246)

Crossword Puzzle

A crossword puzzle grid with the following answers:

- 1 Across: ANGER
- 5 Across: PREVENTION
- 6 Across: MAKEUPPHASE
- 8 Across: TERMINALDISEASE
- 10 Across: EYELEVEL
- 2 Down: EXPLOSIVE
- 3 Down: WITHDRAW
- 4 Down: SMALLNUMBUS (S-M-A-L-L-N-U... M-B-R-S)
- 9 Down: SPEECH
- 7 Down: CID

Critical Thinking

Fill-in-the-Blank

1. situational crisis (page 236)
2. Anger (page 237)
3. Redirection (page 239)
4. empathy (page 239)
5. cries for help (page 244)
6. crowd control (page 240)
7. three (page 240)
8. communicate (page 238)
9. four (page 236)
10. Frustration (page 237)

Short Answer

1. Medical conditions; physical trauma; psychiatric illness; mind-altering substances; and situational stresses (page 236)
2. • Identify yourself and let the patient know you are there to help.
   - Inform the patient of what you are doing.
   - Ask questions in a calm, reassuring voice.
   - Ask the patient to tell you what happened. Do not be judgmental.
   - Show you are listening by using restatement and redirection.
   - Acknowledge the patient's feelings.
   - Assess the patient's mental status through appearance; activity; speech; orientation to person, place, and time; mood; thought process; and memory. (page 240)
3. Perform scene size-up, primary assessment, history taking, secondary assessment, and reassessment. (pages 235–236)
4. You must have a reasonable belief that the patient is going to do harm to himself or herself or to others. (page 243)

5. 1. Working alone or in small numbers

   2. Working late at night or early in the morning

   3. Working in high-crime areas

   4. Working in community settings (page 242)

6. Natural, accidental, and intentional (page 245)

7. Any three of the following:

- Depression
- Inability to sleep
- Weight changes
- Increased alcohol consumption or drug abuse
- Inability to get along with family and coworkers
- Lack of interest in food or sex (page 246)

8. To bring rescuers and a trained person together to talk about rescuers' feelings (page 246)

9. A. "You seem to be worried about getting home to take care of your children. We're going to take good care of you and will make sure your kids are looked after."

   B. "You are very concerned about the woman you hit. My partner is taking care of her now."

   C. "You miss your mommy, don't you? We can go and talk with her as soon as the paramedics finish fixing her leg." (page 239)

10. A. "You seem worried about getting home to take care of your children. Can you give me the name of a friend or neighbor we can call to help take care of them?"

   B. "You are concerned about the woman you hit. My partner is taking care of her, and the paramedics will be here soon. Now we need to examine you to make sure you are not injured."

   C. "You miss your mommy, don't you? When the ambulance gets here, you can ride with your mommy to the hospital. Have you ever been in an ambulance before?" (page 239)

You Make the Call

1. Your answer should include the following steps and information:

- Remain calm.
- Reassure the patient.
- Take time with the patient.
- Make eye contact.
- Touch the patient for reassurance, if appropriate.
- Use a calm and steady voice.
- Use the methods of restatement or redirection to communicate with the patient. (pages 238–239)

2. Your answer should include the following steps and information:

- Obtain a complete history of the incident.
- Determine whether the patient has a weapon or drugs on her.
- Support the patient's ABCs, as needed.
- Dress any open wounds found on the patient.
- Treat the patient for spinal injuries, if suspected.
- Do not judge the patient. Treat her for the injuries or conditions you discover.
- Provide emotional support for the patient and family. (page 244)

Chapter 12: Environmental Emergencies

General Knowledge

Matching

1. C (page 258)
2. H (page 256)
3. F (page 254)
4. B (page 254)
5. E (page 255)
6. A (page 257)
7. G (page 260)
8. D (page 258)

Multiple Choice

1. D (page 255)
2. C (page 254)
3. B (page 257)
4. D (page 257)
5. A (pages 257–258)
6. B (page 254)
7. A (page 255)
8. D (page 256)
9. A (page 257)
10. C (page 257)
11. B (page 258)
12. C (page 260)
13. D (page 260)
14. B (pages 253–254)
15. A (page 260)

True/False

1. T (page 256)
2. F (page 256)
3. T (page 256)
4. F (page 256)
5. T (pages 256–257)
6. T (page 256)
7. F (page 256)
8. T (page 257)
9. F (page 257)
10. T (page 257)
11. F (page 257)
12. T (page 257)
13. T (page 257)
14. T (page 258)
15. T (page 258)
16. T (page 255)
17. F (page 255)
18. T (pages 256–257)
19. T (page 254)
20. F (page 254)
21. T (page 257)
22. F (page 257)
23. T (page 258)
24. T (page 260)
25. F (page 260)

Crossword Puzzle

```
              ¹N O R M A ²L
            ³L           I
            A           G
            R       ⁴E   H
            R       X   T
          ⁵F I N G E R S       ⁶P A N I C
            G       R         I
            O       C         N
            ⁷S H I V E R I N G
            P       S         I
        ⁸C O L D W A T E R D R O W N I N G
            A       S         J
            S             ⁹B A T ¹⁰H T U B
            M             I       R
                          G       Y
                          H
```

Critical Thinking

Fill-in-the-Blank

1. **A.** HE
   B. HE
   C. HS
   D. HE
   E. HS
   F. HS
   G. HE
   H. HE (pages 254–255)
2. cool water (page 254)

3. Drowning (page 258)
4. 30 minutes (page 260)
5. inefficient (page 260)
6. rivers; lakes (page 258)
7. shivering (page 257)
8. rubbing (page 256)
9. groin (page 255)
10. brain damage (page 255)

Fill-in-the-Table (page 255)

Comparing Heat Exhaustion and Heatstroke	
Heat Exhaustion	**Heatstroke**
Normal body temperature	**High** body temperature
Sweating	**Dry** skin (usually)
Cool and **clammy** skin	**Hot** and **red** skin
Dizziness and **nausea**	Semiconscious (or **unconscious**)

Short Answer

1. Face, ears, fingers, and toes (page 256)
2. Light-headedness, dizziness, weak pulse, profuse sweating, and nausea (page 254)
3. • They have decreased sensation to heat and cold.
   • Older bodies are not capable of generating heat as efficiently as younger bodies.
   • Some medications taken by older adults reduce their ability to compensate for hot and cold conditions.
   • Older people tend to drink less fluid, which makes them more susceptible to dehydration. (page 257)
4. • Assess and maintain ABCs.
   • Move the patient from the heat and into a cool place as soon as possible.
   • Remove the patient's clothes, down to the underwear.
   • Soak the patient with water.
   • Place ice packs on the patient's groin.
   • If the patient is conscious and not nauseated, administer small amounts of cool water.
   • Arrange for rapid transport to an appropriate medical facility. (page 255)

You Make the Call

1. Your answer should include the following steps and information:
   • Immediately call for help.
   • Assess scene safety; do not exceed the limits of your training in an attempt to rescue the patient.
   • Perform a primary assessment and establish and correct any airway, breathing, or circulation problems.
   • Be prepared to roll the patient onto his side to allow water to drain out of his mouth.
   • Begin CPR, if indicated.
   • Remove wet clothing from the patient and begin to dry him. Cover the patient as best as possible with a blanket or towel to preserve body temperature.
   • Attempt to obtain any medical information or history.
   • Reassess the patient continuously until additional help arrives.
   • Provide the EMS unit with a complete hand-off report. (page 260)
2. Your answer should include the following steps and information:
   • Complete a scene size-up, including an assessment of scene safety.
   • Conduct a primary assessment of the patient.
   • Immediately move the patient to a cooler area and arrange for transport to a medical facility.
   • Since this patient is conscious, offer him cold water to drink while waiting for EMS.
   • Obtain a SAMPLE history from the patient or bystanders.
   • Perform a secondary assessment, including vital signs.
   • Perform regular reassessments of the patient's ABCs and vital signs while waiting for EMS to arrive. (page 254)

SECTION 5

TRAUMA
Chapter 13: Bleeding, Shock, and Soft-Tissue Injuries

General Knowledge

Matching

1. L (page 282)
2. F (page 283)
3. O (page 282)
4. B (page 282)
5. M (page 286)
6. E (page 282)
7. I (page 294)
8. C (page 273)
9. J (page 283)
10. A (page 282)
11. G (page 294)
12. K (page 282)
13. H (page 270)
14. N (page 295)
15. D (page 271)

Multiple Choice

1. C (page 270)
2. C (page 271)
3. B (page 271)
4. D (page 271)
5. B (page 272)
6. A (page 272)
7. C (page 272)
8. A (pages 272–273)
9. D (page 273)
10. A (page 273)
11. D (page 273)
12. C (page 273)
13. B (page 273)
14. A (page 273)
15. D (page 275)
16. B (page 275)
17. C (page 275)
18. D (page 275)
19. B (pages 275–276)
20. D (page 276)
21. D (page 276)
22. A (pages 292–293)
23. C (pages 290–291)
24. D (page 283)
25. D (page 277)
26. C (page 278)
27. D (page 279)
28. C (page 281)
29. D (page 282)
30. C (page 282)
31. B (page 283)
32. D (page 290)
33. D (page 294)
34. A (page 296)
35. C (page 272)
36. B (page 275)
37. A (page 273)
38. C (page 275)
39. C (page 288)
40. D (page 288)
41. C (page 294)
42. C (page 295)
43. D (pages 296–297)
44. B (page 280)

True/False

1. T (page 271)
2. F (page 271)
3. F (page 271)
4. T (page 271)
5. F (page 272)
6. T (page 272)
7. T (page 270)
8. T (page 273)
9. T (page 274)
10. T (pages 274–275)
11. T (page 275)
12. F (page 275)
13. T (page 275)
14. T (page 276)
15. F (page 282)
16. F (page 284)
17. T (page 273)
18. T (page 289)
19. F (pages 280–281)
20. T (page 279)
21. T (page 282)
22. T (page 283)
23. T (page 288)
24. T (page 289)
25. F (pages 291–292)
26. T (page 275)
27. F (page 275)
28. T (page 289)
29. F (page 290)
30. T (page 283)
31. T (page 298)
32. F (page 298)
33. T (page 297)
34. T (page 298)
35. T (page 289)
36. T (page 280)
37. F (page 279)

Labeling

1. Parts of the Heart
   A. Superior vena cava
   B. Right pulmonary artery
   C. Right atrium
   D. Right ventricle
   E. Inferior vena cava
   F. Aorta
   G. Left pulmonary artery
   H. Left atrium
   I. Pulmonary valve
   J. Left ventricle (page 272)

2. Types of External Bleeding
   A. Venous
   B. Arterial
   C. Capillary (page 278)

3. Types of Wounds
   A. Puncture
   B. Avulsion
   C. Abrasion
   D. Laceration (pages 282–284)

Crossword Puzzle

Across:
4. BRACHIAL ARTERY
7. ENTRANCE WOUND
9. ARTERIAL
11. IV FLUIDS
12. CHF
13. DRESSING
14. ELECTRICAL
15. PSYCHOGENIC

Down:
1. ANAPHYLACTIC
2. SANGUINE (SAI...)
3. CADIORADS
5. ROADSH
6. FEMORAL ARTERY
8. SPLINT
10. RANIBIE

Critical Thinking

Fill-in-the-Blank

1. **A.** 36%
   B. 28%
   C. 18%
   D. 27%
   E. 19% (page 295)

2. **A.** 1
   B. 3
   C. 2
   D. 3
   E. 1
   F. 3
   G. 1
   H. 2
   I. 1, 2
   J. 3 (page 294)

3. tourniquets (page 279)
4. wash; soap; water (pages 281–282)
5. internal (page 282)
6. traumatic (page 283)
7. cleanest (page 283)
8. dressing (page 285)
9. roller gauze; triangular bandages (page 285)
10. secure; slip (page 286)
11. skull fractures; brain injury (page 288)
12. spontaneous (page 288)
13. esophagus; stomach (page 291)
14. bleeding (page 292)
15. patient examination (page 292)
16. infection (page 293)
17. break (page 295)
18. brush away (page 296)
19. pain; injury (page 297)
20. internal; external (page 297)

Short Answer

1. The pump (heart), the pipes (arteries, veins, and capillaries), and the fluid (blood cells and other blood components) (page 271)

2. Pump failure, pipe failure, and fluid loss (page 273)

3. Any three of the following:
   - Clear plastic cover
   - Aluminum foil
   - Plastic wrap
   - Gloves
   - Special dressing that has been impregnated with petroleum jelly (Vaseline™) (page 290)

4. Superficial (first degree), partial thickness (second degree), and full thickness (third degree) (page 294)

5. A dry, sterile dressing or a large sterile cloth called a burn sheet (found in your EMR life support kit) (page 295)

6. Any three of the following:
   - Burns around the face
   - Singed nose hairs
   - Soot in the mouth and nose
   - Difficulty breathing
   - Pain while breathing
   - Unconsciousness as a result of a fire (page 296)

7. 1. Position the patient correctly.
   2. Maintain the patient's ABCs.
   3. Treat the cause of shock, if possible.
   4. Maintain the patient's body temperature by placing blankets under and over the patient.
   5. Make sure the patient does not eat or drink anything.
   6. Assist with other treatments (such as administering oxygen, if available).
   7. Arrange for immediate and prompt transport to an appropriate medical facility. (page 275)

8. 1. Apply a sterile dressing to the wound.
   2. Maintain the patient's body temperature.
   3. Place the patient on his or her back with his or her legs elevated.
   4. Place the patient who is having difficulty breathing in a semireclining position.
   5. Administer oxygen if it is available and if you are trained to use it. (page 291)

9. Control bleeding, prevent further contamination of the wound, immobilize the injured part (reduce or prevent movement), and stabilize any impaled object. (page 284)

You Make the Call

1. Your answer should include the following steps and information:
   - Cool the area with clean, cold water (if available), if the area is still warm.
   - Handle the blistered area carefully.
   - Cover the burned area with dry, sterile dressing or a burn sheet.
   - Remove clothing from the burn site if it is not stuck to the burn.
   - Treat the patient for shock.
   - Arrange for transport to an appropriate medical facility.
   - Complete the head-to-toe physical examination en route. (pages 295–296)

2. Your answer should include the following steps and information:
   - This patient has arterial bleeding.
   - Exert and maintain direct pressure sufficient to stop the bleeding until EMS arrives.
   - Place the patient in a supine position and elevate the extremity.
   - Apply a tourniquet, if permitted and if available.

- If direct pressure and elevation do not stop the bleeding and a tourniquet cannot be used, apply pressure to the brachial pressure point.
- Treat the patient for shock.
- Arrange for prompt transport to an appropriate medical facility. (pages 277–279)

Skills

Skill Drills

Skill Drill 13-1: Controlling Bleeding With a Tourniquet

1. Apply **direct pressure** with a sterile dressing.
2. Apply a **pressure** dressing.
3. If bleeding continues or recurs, apply a tourniquet **above** the level of bleeding. (page 281)

Chapter 14: Injuries to Muscles and Bones

General Knowledge

Matching

1. C (page 308)
2. F (page 309)
3. D (page 309)
4. H (page 309)
5. J (page 325)
6. B (page 307)
7. E (page 319)
8. A (page 328)
9. I (page 319)
10. G (pages 325–326)

Multiple Choice

1. D (page 307)
2. A (page 307)
3. B (page 308)
4. C (page 308)
5. B (page 308)
6. C (pages 308–309)
7. C (page 309)
8. B (page 309)
9. C (page 310)
10. A (page 311)
11. A (page 311)
12. C (page 314)
13. A (page 314)
14. C (page 314)
15. B (page 315)
16. D (pages 325–326, 328)
17. C (page 328)
18. C (page 329)
19. B (page 331)
20. D (pages 335–336)
21. C (page 309)
22. C (page 309)
23. B (page 309)
24. B (page 311)
25. D (page 311)
26. A (page 311)
27. B (page 311)
28. C (page 311)
29. B (page 314)
30. C (page 315)
31. C (page 320)
32. D (page 320)
33. C (page 310)
34. A (page 318)
35. A (page 330)
36. B (pages 336–337)

True/False

1. T (page 306)
2. T (page 307)
3. T (page 307)
4. T (page 307)
5. F (page 309)
6. F (page 310)
7. T (page 311)
8. F (page 311)
9. T (page 310)
10. F (pages 313–314)
11. T (page 314)
12. F (page 314)
13. F (page 314)
14. T (page 315)
15. F (page 319)
16. T (page 319)
17. T (page 320)
18. F (page 326)
19. T (page 326)
20. T (page 329)
21. F (page 329)
22. T (page 331)
23. F (page 331)
24. T (page 331)
25. T (page 310)
26. T (page 310)
27. T (page 310)
28. F (page 310)
29. F (page 314)
30. F (page 314)
31. F (page 314)
32. T (page 319)
33. T (page 319)
34. T (page 319)
35. T (page 336)
36. T (page 309)
37. F (page 334)

Labeling

1. The Human Skeleton
   A. Head
   B. Spinal column
   C. Shoulder girdle
   D. Upper extremity
   E. Rib cage
   F. Pelvis
   G. Lower extremity (page 306)
   D. Sacrum
   E. Coccyx (page 307)

2. Sections of the Spine
   A. Cervical
   B. Thoracic
   C. Lumbar

3. Types of Muscle
   A. Cardiac muscle
   B. Skeletal muscle
   C. Smooth muscle (page 308)

Crossword Puzzle

Critical Thinking

Fill-in-the-Blank

1. rigid collar (page 331)
2. obstruction (page 329)
3. mechanism (page 308)
4. dislocation (page 309)
5. Battle's (page 328)

6. abdominal (page 331)
7. flail (page 335)
8. Osteoporosis (page 319)
9. CPR (page 331)
10. traction (page 314)

Short Answer

1. Support the body, protect vital structures, assist in body movement, and manufacture red blood cells (page 306)
2. Fractures, dislocations, and sprains (page 309)
3. Open wound, deformity, swelling, and bruising (page 310)
4. "Where does it hurt most?" and "Is it numb or tingling?" (page 310)
5. Pulse and capillary refill (page 311)
6. Any three of the following:
   - Laceration, bruise, or other sign of injury to the head, neck, or spine
   - Tenderness over any point on spine or neck
   - Pain in the neck or spine or pain radiating to an extremity
   - Extremity weakness, numbness, paralysis, or loss of movement
   - Loss of sensation or movement, tingling/burning sensation in any part of the body below the neck
   - Loss of bowel or bladder control (page 331)

7. Pulse, capillary refill, sensation, and movement distal to the point of injury (page 314)
8. 1. Support and stabilize the injured limb.
   2. Form the SAM splint to the injured forearm.
   3. Place the splint under the injured limb.
   4. Secure the splint in place with gauze.
   5. Recheck the pulse, capillary refill, and sensation of the injured forearm. (page 316)
9. 1. **Direct force**: A car strikes a pedestrian on the leg. The pedestrian sustains a broken leg.
   2. **Indirect force**: A woman falls on her shoulder. The force of the fall transmits energy to the middle of the collarbone, and the excess force breaks the bone.
   3. **Twisting force**: A football player is tackled as he is turning. As the leg twists, the knee sustains a severe injury. (page 308)
10. 1. Head, skull, and face
    2. Spinal column
    3. Shoulder girdle
    4. Upper extremities
    5. Rib cage (thorax)
    6. Pelvis
    7. Lower extremities (page 306)
11. • Splint the elbow joint in the position it was found in.
    • If the patient does not have a significant shoulder injury (and only if it does not cause pain), gently move the splinted injury to the patient's side for comfort and ease of transport. (page 316)
12. Any four of the following:
    • Confusion
    • Unusual behavior
    • Unconsciousness
    • Nausea or vomiting
    • Blood from an ear
    • Decreasing consciousness
    • Unequal pupils
    • Paralysis
    • Seizures
    • Raccoon eyes
    • Battle's sign
    • External head trauma (bleeding, bumps, contusions) (page 328)
13. Immobilize the head in a neutral position, maintain an open airway, support the patient's breathing, monitor circulation, assess for CSF or blood seeping from the nose or ears, control any bleeding from all head wounds with dry and sterile dressings, examine and treat any other serious injuries, and arrange for prompt transport to an appropriate medical facility. (pages 328–329)
14. Any three of the following:
    • Pain at the injury site
    • An open wound
    • Swelling and discoloration (bruising)
    • The patient's inability or unwillingness to move the extremity
    • Deformity or angulation
    • Tenderness at the injury site (page 310)

You Make the Call

1. Your answer should include the following steps and information:
   - Determine the mechanism of injury.
   - Conduct a general patient assessment.
   - Stabilize the patient's airway, breathing, and circulation.
   - Examine the injured leg.
   - Evaluate circulation, sensation, and movement in the leg.
   - Provide treatment (including proper steps for bandaging and splinting). (pages 308–325)

2. Your answer should include the following steps and information:
   - Establish scene safety and apply standard precautions.
   - Immobilize the patient's head in a neutral position.
   - Assess and verify that airway, breathing, and circulation are adequate.
   - Consider applying oxygen to the patient.
   - Assess for any CSF or blood seeping from the nose or ears.
   - Control external bleeding with dry, sterile dressings.
   - Perform a detailed assessment and treat other serious injuries.
   - Arrange for prompt transport to an appropriate medical facility. (pages 325–329)

Skills

Skill Drills

Skill Drill 14-1: Checking Circulation, Sensation, and Movement in an Injured Extremity

1. Check for circulation. If upper extremity injury, check **radial** pulse.
2. If lower extremity injury, check **posterior tibial** pulse.
3. Test **capillary refill** on finger/toe of injured limb.
4. Release pressure. **Pink** color should return.
5. Check for **sensation** at fingertips.
6. Check for **sensation** at toes.
7. Check for **movement** of the upper extremities by asking the patient to open and close the fist.
8. Check for **movement** of the lower extremities by asking the patient to extend and flex the ankle. (pages 312–313)

Skill Drill 14-4: Applying a Traction Splint

1. Place the splint beside the **uninjured** limb, adjust the splint to the proper length, and prepare the straps.
2. Support the injured limb as your partner fastens the **ankle hitch** about the foot and ankle.
3. Continue to support the limb as your partner applies gentle **traction** to the **ankle hitch** and foot.
4. Slide the **splint** into position under the injured limb.
5. Pad the **groin** and fasten the strap around the **midthigh**.
6. Connect the loops of the ankle hitch to the end of the splint as your partner continues to maintain **traction**. Fasten the support straps so that the **limb** is securely held in the splint. (page 322)

Skill Drill 14-8: Removing the Mask on a Sports Helmet

1. Stabilize the patient's head and helmet in a **neutral**, in-line position. Then remove the mask in one of the following two ways.
2. Use a **screwdriver** to unscrew the retaining clips for the face mask or perform Step 3.
3. Use a **trainer's tool** designed for cutting retaining clips. (page 333)

Skill Drill 14-9: Removing a Helmet

1. Kneel down at the patient's head and open the face shield to assess the **airway** and **breathing**. Stabilize the helmet by placing your hands on either side of it, ensuring that your fingers are on the patient's **lower jaw** to prevent movement of the head. Your partner can then loosen the strap.

2. Your partner should place one hand on the patient's **lower jaw** and the other behind the **head** at the occiput.

3. Gently slip the helmet off about **halfway** and then stop.

4. Your partner slides his or her hand from the occiput to the **back** of the head to prevent the head from snapping back once the helmet is removed.

5. With your partner's hand in place, remove the helmet and stabilize the **cervical spine**. Apply a cervical collar and then secure the patient to a long backboard. (pages 334–335)

Chapter 15: Childbirth

General Knowledge

Matching

1. E (page 345)	**3.** H (page 345)	**5.** I (page 345)	**7.** C (pages 350–351)	**9.** J (page 345)
2. G (page 354)	**4.** B (page 346)	**6.** A (page 345)	**8.** F (page 346)	**10.** D (page 356)

Multiple Choice

1. B (page 346)	**7.** A (page 347)	**13.** C (page 354)	**19.** B (page 351)	**24.** C (page 354)
2. B (pages 354, 356)	**8.** A (page 348)	**14.** C (page 345)	**20.** C (page 356)	**25.** A (page 354)
3. C (page 346)	**9.** D (page 346)	**15.** B (page 345)	**21.** D (pages 350, 352–353)	**26.** B (page 347)
4. D (pages 346–347)	**10.** B (page 350)	**16.** A (page 346)		**27.** D (page 357)
5. A (page 346)	**11.** D (page 350)	**17.** B (page 346)	**22.** B (page 347)	
6. C (page 347)	**12.** D (page 356)	**18.** D (page 348)	**23.** D (page 352)	

True/False

1. F (page 348)	**7.** F (pages 354, 356)	**13.** T (page 346)	**19.** F (page 348)	**25.** T (page 354)
2. T (page 348)	**8.** F (page 357)	**14.** T (page 346)	**20.** F (page 348)	**26.** T (page 357)
3. F (page 350)	**9.** T (page 354)	**15.** F (page 347)	**21.** F (page 348)	**27.** F (page 357)
4. F (page 350)	**10.** F (page 356)	**16.** F (page 346)	**22.** F (page 350)	**28.** F (page 357)
5. F (page 356)	**11.** F (pages 345–346)	**17.** T (page 347)	**23.** T (page 352)	
6. F (page 356)	**12.** F (page 346)	**18.** T (page 348)	**24.** F (page 352)	

Labeling

1. **Anatomy of a Pregnant Woman**
   - **A.** Placenta
   - **B.** Uterus
   - **C.** Amniotic fluid
   - **D.** Sacrum
   - **E.** Rectum
   - **F.** Bladder
   - **G.** Vagina (page 346)

2. **Phases of the Second Stage of Labor**
   - **A.** Head begins to deliver
   - **B.** Delivery of head
   - **C.** Delivery of upper shoulder
   - **D.** Delivery of lower shoulder (page 350)

Crossword Puzzle

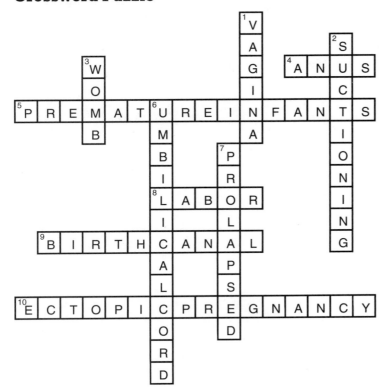

Critical Thinking

Fill-in-the-Blank

1. placenta (page 345)
2. one (page 346)
3. crowning (page 347)
4. assist (page 348)
5. umbilical (page 350)
6. breech (page 356)
7. miscarriage (page 354)
8. multiple (page 356)
9. beginning (page 347)
10. premature (page 354)

Short Answer

1. **Stage one**: Initial contractions occur, bag of waters breaks, bloody show occurs (mucus plug), no crowning occurs
   Stage two: Crowning of the infant's head occurs, followed by birth of the infant
   Stage three: Delivery of placenta occurs (page 346)
2. 1. Is this the woman's first pregnancy?
   2. Has the woman experienced a bloody show?
   3. Has the bag of waters broken?
   4. How frequent are the contractions?
   5. Does the woman feel an urge to move her bowels?
   6. Is the infant's head crowning?
   7. Is transportation available? (pages 345–346)
3. 1. Carefully open the sterile glove package without touching the gloves.
   2. Pick up the first glove by grasping one edge.
   3. Pull on the first glove, being careful not to touch the outside of the glove.

    4. Grasp the second glove by sliding two fingers of your hand into the rolled edge.

    5. Put on the second glove.

    6. Keep the gloves as sterile as possible. (page 348)

4. Any three of the following:

- Save the fetus and tissues that pass from the vagina to transport with the patient.
- Control bleeding.
- Treat for shock.
- Arrange for prompt transport to an appropriate medical facility.
- Provide emotional support to the patient and her family. (page 354)

You Make the Call

1. Your answer should include the following steps and information:

- Determine whether or not the bloody show has occurred.
- Determine whether or not the bag of waters has broken.
- Assess the frequency of contractions.
- Ask the woman if she feels the urge to move her bowels.
- Determine if the infant's head is crowning.
- Either arrange for transport or prepare for delivery.
- Calm and reassure the patient. (pages 346–347)

2. Your answer should include the following steps and information:

- It is possible this woman is experiencing an ectopic pregnancy. Any woman of childbearing age who presents with severe abdominal pain or signs and symptoms of shock needs to be evaluated for a possible rupture of an ectopic pregnancy.
- Your treatment begins with a complete patient assessment, including a SAMPLE history.
- Be sure to measure the patient's vital signs.
- Treat the patient for shock and arrange for prompt transport to an appropriate medical facility. (page 354)

Skills

Skill Drills

Skill Drill 15-2: Resuscitating a Newborn

    1. Tilt the infant so the **head** is down and to the side to clear the airway.

    2. Gently snap or flick your fingers on the **soles** of the infant's feet.

    3. Begin **rescue breathing**.

    4. Check for a **brachial** pulse.

    5. Begin **chest compressions** using the middle and ring fingers. (page 353)

Chapter 16: Pediatric Emergencies

General Knowledge

Matching

1. C (page 377)
2. B (page 367)
3. F (page 370)
4. E (page 379)
5. D (page 376)
6. G (page 376)
7. A (page 377)

Multiple Choice

1. A (page 369)
2. B (page 372)
3. A (page 383)
4. B (page 383)
5. C (page 384)
6. A (page 375)
7. B (page 376)
8. C (page 369)
9. B (page 367)
10. B (page 366)
11. C (page 366)
12. D (page 366)
13. C (page 368)
14. A (page 368)
15. A (page 368)
16. C (page 368)
17. C (page 374)
18. D (page 370)
19. B (page 372)
20. D (page 375)
21. A (page 374)
22. D (page 374)
23. D (page 375)
24. C (page 377)
25. B (page 377)
26. C (page 377)
27. D (page 379)
28. B (page 379)
29. A (page 379)
30. C (page 381)
31. A (page 379)
32. D (page 382)
33. A (page 383)
34. C (pages 364–365)
35. B (page 365)

True/False

1. T (page 364)
2. T (page 365)
3. F (page 365)
4. T (pages 379, 381)
5. F (page 381)
6. T (page 381)
7. F (page 378)
8. T (page 379)
9. T (page 378)
10. T (page 378)
11. T (page 382)
12. F (page 383)
13. T (page 382)
14. F (page 382)
15. T (page 371)
16. T (pages 371–372)
17. F (page 372)
18. T (pages 377–378)
19. T (page 368)
20. F (page 368)
21. F (page 369)
22. F (page 370)
23. F (page 365)
24. T (page 374)
25. T (page 374)
26. F (pages 375–376)
27. F (page 376)
28. T (page 376)
29. F (page 376)
30. T (page 377)
31. F (page 377)
32. T (page 379)
33. T (page 379)
34. T (page 379)
35. F (page 381)
36. T (page 366)
37. T (page 382)
38. F (page 384)

Crossword Puzzle

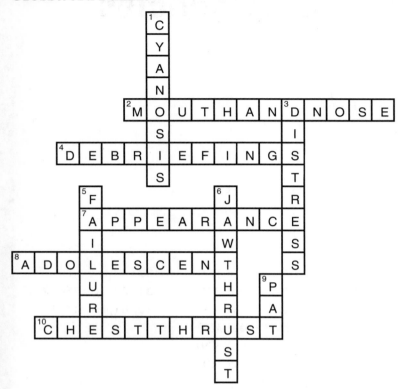

Critical Thinking

Fill-in-the-Blank

1. 3 weeks; 7 months (page 381)
2. Pallor (page 367)
3. pediatric assessment triangle (page 366)
4. 90 to 180; 30 to 60 (page 368)
5. trauma (page 382)

6. mild (partial); back; chin (page 371)
7. 1 year (page 376)
8. Drowning (page 377)
9. heatstroke (page 378)
10. dehydration (page 379)

Short Answer

1. 1. Respirations
   2. Pulse rate
   3. Body temperature (page 368)
2. Sharp or straight objects such as:
   1. Open safety pins
   2. Bobby pins
   3. Bones (page 374)

3. **1.** Open and maintain the airway.

   2. Control bleeding.

   3. Arrange for prompt transport to an appropriate medical facility. (page 383)

4. **1.** Remove the child's clothing.

   2. Sponge water over the child.

   3. Fan the child to help lower the body temperature quickly.

   4. Wrap the child in wet sheets (if they are available) to speed up the evaporation and cooling process.

   5. Make sure the child does not become chilled.

   6. Arrange for rapid transport to an appropriate medical facility. (page 378)

5. **1.** Make certain the child is not wrapped in too much clothing or too many blankets.

   2. Attempt to reduce the high temperature by undressing the child.

   3. Fan the child to cool him or her down.

   4. Protect the child during any seizure (do not restrain the child's motion), and make certain that normal breathing resumes after each seizure. (page 379)

6. Treat every child with a sore or tender abdomen as an emergency and arrange for transport to an appropriate medical facility for an appropriate diagnosis. (page 379)

7. **1.** Lack of adult supervision

   2. Malnourished-appearing child

   3. Unsafe living environment

   4. Untreated chronic illness (page 384)

8. Summon law enforcement personnel and explain your concerns to them. (page 384)

9. If the infant is still warm (page 381)

You Make the Call

1. Your answer should include the following steps and information:

- Be alert for injuries to the chest, abdomen, legs, and head.
- Check the patient's ABCs.
- Control severe bleeding and treat the patient for shock.
- Perform a full-body assessment.
- Stabilize all injuries.
- Keep the child warm.
- Give oxygen, if available.
- Arrange for immediate transport to an appropriate medical facility. (pages 382–383)

2. Your answer should include the following steps and information:

- Call for assistance and verify EMS was dispatched.
- Consider a possible cervical spine injury, and stabilize the neck.
- Assess airway, breathing, and circulation.
- Make sure the airway is clear of water. Turn the child to one side and allow the water to drain out of the mouth. Use suction, if it is available.
- Begin rescue breathing and provide supplemental oxygen with a bag-mask device, if available.
- If there is no pulse, begin chest compressions.
- Cover the child with blankets to maintain body heat and prevent hypothermia. (pages 377–378)

Skills

Skill Drills

Skill Drill 16-1: Inserting an Oral Airway in a Child

1. Select the proper size oral airway by measuring from the patient's **earlobe** to the corner of the **mouth**.

2. **Position** the pediatric patient's airway with the appropriate method.

3. Depress the patient's tongue and press the tongue **forward** and away from the **roof** of the mouth. Follow the anatomic curve of the roof of the patient's mouth to **slide** the airway into place. (page 371)

Chapter 17: Geriatric Emergencies

General Knowledge

Matching

1. B (page 400)
2. D (page 395)
3. A (page 400)
4. C (page 401)
5. F (page 400)
6. G (page 400)
7. E (page 400)

Multiple Choice

1. A (page 395)
2. D (page 395)
3. C (pages 393–394)
4. A (page 394)
5. D (page 395)
6. D (page 393)
7. D (page 393)
8. B (page 393)
9. A (page 395)
10. C (page 395)
11. B (page 396)
12. A (page 398)

True/False

1. T (page 398)
2. F (page 394)
3. F (page 393)
4. T (page 395)
5. F (page 394)
6. T (page 395)
7. T (page 401)
8. T (page 394)
9. T (page 398)
10. F (page 399)
11. T (page 398)
12. T (page 394)
13. F (page 394)
14. T (page 398)
15. T (page 398)
16. T (page 395)
17. F (page 399)
18. F (page 396)
19. T (page 400)
20. T (page 400)
21. F (page 402)
22. F (page 401)
23. T (pages 401–402)
24. T (page 401)
25. F (page 400)

Labeling

1. Simple Phrases in Sign Language
   A. Sick
   B. Help
   C. Hurt (page 394)

Crossword Puzzle

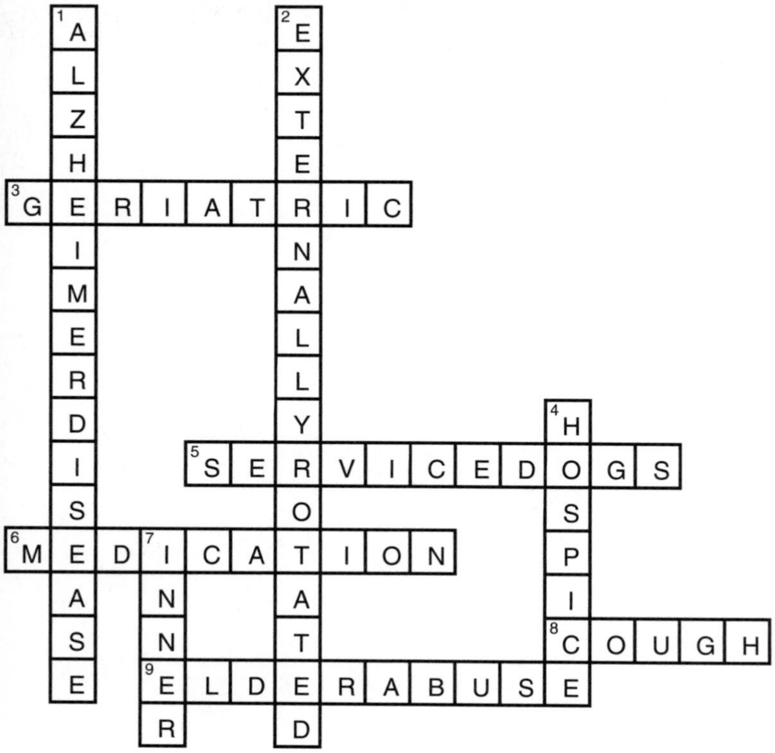
1 ALZHEIMERDISEASE
2 EXTERNALLYROTATED
3 GERIATRIC
4 HOSPICE
5 SERVICEDOGS
6 MEDICATION
7 INNER
8 COUGH
9 ELDERABUSE

Critical Thinking

Fill-in-the-Blank

1. more (page 393)
2. bladder (page 394)
3. Hearing loss (page 394)
4. Fractures (page 395)
5. medications (page 398)
6. hospice (page 401)
7. Osteoporosis (page 395)
8. Alzheimer disease (page 400)
9. shortened (page 396)
10. acute (page 396)
11. Pneumonia (page 396)
12. Catheters (page 399)

Fill-in-the-Table (page 396)

Disabilities That May Occur With Age
• **Hearing** loss or impairment
• Sight **loss** or impairment
• Loss of **sensation**
• **Slowed** movements
• **Fractures**
• Senility
• Loss of **bowel** or **bladder** control

Short Answer

1. **1.** The injured leg is usually (but not always) shortened as compared with the other leg.
   2. The toes of the injured leg are externally rotated.
   3. The pain may be so great that the patient cannot move the injured leg. (page 396)

2. Any three of the following:
   - Identify yourself.
   - Look directly at the patient.
   - Speak slowly and distinctly.
   - Explain what you are going to do in clear, simple language.
   - Listen to the patient.
   - Show the patient respect.
   - Do not talk about the patient in front of the patient.
   - Be patient. (page 395)

3. Any three of the following:
   - Bruises, especially on the buttocks, lower back, genitals, cheeks, neck, and earlobes
   - Pressure bruises caused by a human hand
   - Multiple bruises in different states of healing
   - Burns
   - Trauma in the genital area
   - Signs of neglect, such as malnourished appearance (page 402)

4. Any three of the following:
   - Physical illnesses
   - Loss of a loved one
   - Alcohol abuse
   - Hopelessness
   - Depression
   - Previous suicide attempts (page 400)

You Make the Call

1. Your answer should include the following steps and information:
   - Speak clearly and calmly to the patient.
   - Find out what medications the patient is taking and what was taken when.
   - Arrange for transport to the hospital.
   - Gather up the patient's medications and bring them to the hospital.
   - Let the patient know what you are doing at each step of your assessment.
   - Ask family members or caregivers for a medical history.
   - Try to avoid asking the patient if it is all right to do something; instead, gently inform her of the treatment. (pages 398, 401)

2. Your answer should include the following steps and information:
   - Assess the patient for any signs of life-threatening conditions (eg, airway complications, internal hemorrhaging).
   - Verify that EMS was dispatched and is responding.
   - Obtain a thorough history and keep in mind possible medical causes for the fall (eg, stroke, heart attack, confusion).
   - Assess pulse, motor, and sensation in the foot to note any compromise to the circulation or nerves in the extremity.
   - Immobilize the hip in the position it was found in. Use several pillows or rolled blankets, especially under the flexed knee.
   - Place the patient on a long backboard (if available) in preparation for transport.
   - Reassess pulse, motor, and sensation after the splint is applied.
   - Obtain a set of vital signs and perform a head-to-toe physical examination, while remaining alert for any other injuries from the fall. (pages 319, 395–396)

EMS OPERATIONS
Chapter 18: Lifting and Moving Patients

General Knowledge

Matching

1. C (page 413)   **4.** D (page 413)   **7.** A (page 425)   **10.** I (pages 414–415)
2. H (page 413)   **5.** B (page 425)   **8.** G (page 418)
3. J (pages 412–413)   **6.** F (page 412)   **9.** E (pages 421–422)

Multiple Choice

1. C (pages 425, 427)   **6.** D (page 425)   **11.** A (page 418)   **16.** D (pages 415–416)
2. D (pages 412–413)   **7.** C (page 428)   **12.** A (pages 414–415)   **17.** C (page 421)
3. C (page 413)   **8.** B (page 421)   **13.** C (page 415)   **18.** B (page 419)
4. B (page 413)   **9.** D (pages 421–422)   **14.** D (page 415)   **19.** A (page 423)
5. D (pages 425, 427)   **10.** A (page 423)   **15.** B (page 415)   **20.** C (page 412)

True/False

1. F (page 414)   **10.** T (page 421)   **19.** F (page 423)   **28.** T (page 411)
2. T (page 416)   **11.** F (page 421)   **20.** F (page 423)   **29.** F (page 411)
3. F (page 416)   **12.** T (page 421)   **21.** T (page 425)   **30.** T (page 412)
4. T (page 417)   **13.** F (pages 421–422)   **22.** T (pages 425, 427)   **31.** T (page 414)
5. F (page 418)   **14.** T (page 422)   **23.** F (pages 427–428)   **32.** T (page 414)
6. T (page 418)   **15.** F (page 422)   **24.** F (page 428)   **33.** T (page 414)
7. T (page 419)   **16.** F (page 422)   **25.** F (page 431)   **34.** T (page 412)
8. F (page 419)   **17.** F (page 422)   **26.** T (page 411)   **35.** T (page 412)
9. T (page 421)   **18.** F (page 423)   **27.** T (page 411)

Labeling

1. Carries and Drags

   A. Arm-to-arm drag (page 414)
   B. Two-person walking assist (page 419)
   C. Two-person extremity carry (page 415)
   D. Cradle-in-arms carry (page 416)
   E. Two-person seat carry (page 415)
   F. Blanket drag (page 413)

   G. One-person walking assist (page 418)
   H. Pack-strap carry (page 416)
   I. Emergency clothes drag (page 413)
   J. Two-person chair carry (page 416)
   K. Fire fighter drag (page 414)

Crossword Puzzle

Across/grid answers:

- 1 PACKSTRAP
- 3 CHAIRCARRY
- 5 WALKINGASSIST
- 6 SEATCARRY
- 7 STAIRCHAIR
- 8 STRADDLESLIDE

Down entries include: PORTABLETABLE, CRADLEINARMS, CERVICALCOLLAR, EXTREMITIE, WALKINGASSIST, STRETCHER, EXTREMITIES.

Critical Thinking

Fill-in-the-Blank

1. log rolling (page 425)
2. immobilize (page 421)
3. Cervical collars (page 422)
4. scoop (pages 421–422)
5. Soft (page 422)
6. head (page 425)
7. four (page 425)
8. portable stretcher (page 421)
9. direct ground lift (page 416)
10. improvise (page 431)

Short Answer

1. For the protection of the patient; if rescuers need more room to provide treatment (page 411)
2. Keep the patient's head and spine immobilized so he or she does not move. (page 411)
3. To help maintain an open airway and allow secretions to drain from the patient's mouth (page 412)
4. Any three of the following:
   - There is danger of fire, explosion, or structural collapse.
   - Hazardous materials are present.
   - The accident scene cannot be protected.
   - It is otherwise impossible to gain access to other patients who need lifesaving care.
   - The patient has experienced cardiac arrest and must be moved so that you can begin CPR. (pages 412)

5. Any three of the following:
- Wheeled ambulance stretcher
- Portable stretcher
- Stair chair
- Long backboard
- Short backboard (vest-type immobilizer)
- Scoop stretcher (page 419)

6. 1. Do no further harm to the patient.
   2. Move the patient only when necessary.
   3. Move the patient as little as possible.
   4. Move the patient's body as a unit.
   5. Use proper lifting and moving techniques to ensure your own safety.
   6. Have one rescuer give commands when moving a patient (usually the rescuer at the patient's head). (page 411)

7. Any three of the following:
- Wide, sturdy planks
- Doors
- Ironing boards
- Sturdy folding tables
- Full-length lawn chair recliners
- Surfboards
- Snowboards (page 422)

You Make the Call

1. In this situation, you will want to use one of the following techniques to remove this patient from the hazardous environment:

Two-person walking assist:
   1. Help the patient stand.
   2. Have the patient place one arm around your neck and hold the patient's wrist, which should be draped over your shoulder. Put your free arm around the patient's waist and help the patient walk.
   3. Have the patient do the same with the other rescuer.
   4. Two rescuers can support the patient as they escort him from his home.

Two-person chair carry:
   1. Rescuer One stands behind the seated patient, reaches down, and grasps the back of the chair close to the seat.
   2. Rescuer One then tilts the chair slightly backward on its rear legs so that Rescuer Two can step back in between the legs of the chair and grasp the chair's front legs.
   3. The patient's legs should be between the legs of the chair.
   4. When both rescuers are correctly positioned, Rescuer One gives the command to lift and walk away.

Two-person seat carry:
   1. The rescuers kneel on opposite sides of the patient near the patient's hips.
   2. The rescuers then raise the patient to a sitting position and link arms behind the patient's back.
   3. The rescuers then place their other arm under the patient's knees and link with each other.
   4. If possible, the patient should put his arms around the necks and shoulders of the rescuers for additional support. (pages 415, 418)

2. Your answer should include the following steps and information:

- Because this patient presents with no potential life-threatening conditions, a short backboard device can be used to immobilize the patient.
- One of the providers should go behind the patient to stabilize the head, while the other responder places a cervical collar on the patient.
- While maintaining neutral, in-line motion restriction, lean the patient forward while a responder slides the device behind the patient, head first.
- Carefully lean the patient against the board.
- Fasten the middle strap of the device, and then fasten the rest of the straps.
- Place the wings of the device around the patient's head and strap the patient's head to the device.
- Carefully move the patient from the vehicle and place her on a long backboard (if available) while waiting for EMS to arrive. (pages 423–425)

Skills

Skill Drills

Skill Drill 18-3: Four-Person Log Roll

1. Rescuers get into position to **roll** the patient.
2. Roll the patient onto his or her **side**.
3. The fourth person slides the **backboard** toward the patient.
4. **Roll** the patient onto the backboard.
5. Center the patient on the backboard and **secure** the patient before moving. (page 426)

Skill Drill 18-5: Applying the Blanket Roll to Stabilize the Patient's Head and Neck

1. **Stabilize** the head.
2. Apply a **cervical collar**.
3. Place the **straps** around the backboard and patient.
4. Insert the **blanket roll** and roll each side of the blanket snugly against the **neck** and shoulders.
5. Tie two **cravats** around the blanket roll, then two more around the blanket roll and backboard. (page 430)

Chapter 19: Transport Operations

General Knowledge

Matching

1. A (page 437)
2. H (pages 437–438)
3. C, J (pages 438–439)
4. D, F, I (page 439)
5. G (page 439)
6. B, E (page 439)

Multiple Choice

1. A (page 437)
2. C (page 438)
3. B (pages 438–439)
4. D (page 439)
5. C (page 439)
6. A (page 439)
7. B (page 441)
8. D (page 441)
9. C (page 441)
10. A (page 441)

True/False

1. T (page 437)
2. T (page 437)
3. F (page 438)
4. T (page 438)
5. F (page 438)
6. F (page 438)
7. T (page 439)
8. T (page 439)
9. T (page 441)
10. F (page 441)

Crossword Puzzle

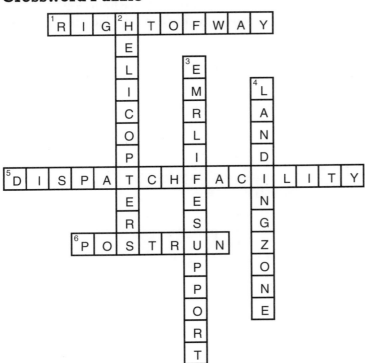

Critical Thinking

Fill-in-the-Blank

1. dispatch facilities (page 437)
2. missile (page 438)
3. bystanders (page 439)
4. Helicopters (page 441)
5. Fusees (page 441)

Short Answer

1. 1. Be alert for electrical wires when identifying a landing zone for a helicopter.
    2. Always approach helicopters from the front so the pilot can see you. Approaching a helicopter from the rear is dangerous because the tail rotor is nearly invisible when spinning.
    3. Do not approach the helicopter until the pilot signals that it is safe to do so.
    4. Helicopters are very noisy and you may not be able to hear a shouted warning. Maintain eye contact with the pilot.
    5. Keep low when you approach the helicopter to avoid the spinning main rotor blades.
    6. Follow the directions of the helicopter crew. (page 441)
2. • DO NOT approach the helicopter landing zone unless necessary.
    • DO NOT approach a helicopter from the upside if it is on a slope.
    • DO NOT run near a helicopter.
    • DO NOT raise your hand when approaching a helicopter. (page 442)

You Make the Call

1. Your answer should include the following steps and information:
    • Contact your dispatch center or directly contact the helicopter dispatch center to request a helicopter. Follow your local guidelines.
    • Determine the safest area near the scene to set up a landing zone. Make sure the area is level, free from electrical wires and trees, and there is plenty of room. If there are potential hazards in the area, have the dispatch center communicate those to the pilot.
    • Mark an area of at least 100′ × 100′ with clearly visible markers that are safe and do not distract the pilot.
    • Make sure the area is clear of debris. Close the windows and doors of nearby vehicles and remove any loose objects on the vehicles that could become airborne.
    • Depending on your local guidelines, consider having the fire department standing by with a charged hose line. (page 441)
2. Your answer should include the following steps and information:
    • Place your vehicle in a safe location to minimize the chance of injury.
    • Perform a scene size-up before you exit the vehicle.
    • Identify hazards, such as downed electrical lines, leaking fuel, broken glass, and fires.
    • Control the flow of traffic to ensure safety to rescuers, patients, and bystanders.
    • Determine the number of patients, and determine whether you need additional resources. (page 439)

Chapter 20: Vehicle Extrication and Special Rescue

General Knowledge

Matching

1. D (page 460)
2. J (page 458)
3. I (page 457)
4. A (page 458)
5. F (page 460)
6. H (page 450)
7. G (page 449)
8. B (page 447)
9. E (page 452)
10. C (page 448)

Multiple Choice

1. D (page 458)
2. D (page 458)
3. C (page 460)
4. A (page 461)
5. B (page 458)
6. A (pages 459–460)
7. A (page 460)
8. B (page 460)
9. D (page 460)
10. C (page 461)
11. B (page 464)
12. D (page 448)
13. A (page 448)
14. D (page 449)
15. C (page 451)
16. C (page 452)
17. B (page 454)
18. C (page 455)
19. A (page 463)
20. A (page 461)

True/False

1. T (page 460)
2. F (page 458)
3. T (page 458)
4. T (pages 458–459)
5. T (page 458)
6. F (page 459)
7. F (page 464)
8. F (page 457)
9. T (page 452)
10. T (page 454)
11. T (page 463)
12. F (page 461)
13. F (page 458)
14. T (page 458)
15. F (page 458)
16. T (page 460)
17. F (page 460)
18. F (page 465)
19. T (page 461)
20. T (page 461)
21. T (page 448)
22. F (page 449)
23. T (page 450)
24. T (page 450)
25. F (page 451)

Crossword Puzzle

```
                              ¹C
                         ²G   R
   ³E X ⁴T R I C A T I   O    N
      H      S           B
 ⁵R E S C U E T H R O W  B A  ⁶G
      B          L       I    O
      E          I       N    L
      N          N       G    D
 ⁷D O W N E D W I R E S       E
      S          S            N
                 P            P
   ⁸I ⁹M P A C T F I R E      E
      A          L            R
      R          L            I
      K                       O
                              D
```

Critical Thinking

Fill-in-the-Blank

1. flotation (page 458)
2. row (page 457)
3. airway (page 458)
4. head; neck (page 458)
5. air; decompression sickness (the bends) (page 460)
6. oxygen (page 461)
7. delayed (page 461)
8. Riptides (page 458)
9. jump (page 457)
10. cardiac arrest (page 458)
11. unstable; stabilized (page 450)
12. fire (page 455)
13. Golden Period (page 456)
14. extrication (page 456)
15. gain access (page 452)

Short Answer

1. 1. Reach
   2. Throw
   3. Row
   4. Go (pages 457–458)
2. Any three of the following:
   - Dizziness
   - Difficulty speaking
   - Difficulty seeing
   - Decreased level of consciousness
   - Difficulty maintaining an open airway
   - Chest pain
   - Shortness of breath
   - Pink or bloody froth coming from the mouth or nose
   - Severe abdominal pain
   - Joint pain (page 460)
3. Any five of the following:
   - Manholes
   - Below-ground utility vaults
   - Below-ground or ground-level storage tanks
   - Old mines
   - Cisterns
   - Wells
   - Industrial tankers
   - Farm storage silos
   - Water towers (page 461)
4. Respiratory hazards (including insufficient oxygen or poisonous gases); danger of collapse (page 461)
5. 1. Conduct an overview of the scene.
   2. Stabilize the scene, control any hazards, and stabilize the vehicle.
   3. Gain access to patients.
   4. Provide initial emergency care.
   5. Help disentangle patients.
   6. Help prepare patients for removal.
   7. Help remove patients. (page 448)

You Make the Call

1. Your answer should include the following steps and information:
   - Carefully overview the scene to determine the scope of the problem.
   - Treat the silo as a confined space and do not enter without proper self-contained breathing apparatus and proper training.
   - Call for adequate assistance from fire, rescue, and EMS organizations.
   - If possible, gain access to the patient.
   - Provide initial emergency care to the patient, including establishing responsiveness, supporting the patient's ABCs, controlling bleeding, and maintaining the patient's body temperature.
   - Talk with the patient and provide psychological support.
   - As other rescuers arrive on the scene, help them to disentangle the patient, prepare the patient for removal, and remove the patient. (pages 461, 463–464)

2. Your answer should include the following steps and information:

- Immediately call for assistance from fire, rescue, and EMS services.
- Use your dry chemical fire extinguisher to keep the flames out of the passenger compartment by directing the extinguisher to the base of the fire.
- Immediately have someone else gather fire extinguishers from other vehicles present on the scene. This is in case your extinguisher runs out before the fire is extinguished.
- Remove the patients as quickly as possible, but take care because they may have sustained injuries from the crash.
- Move everyone at least 50 feet away from the vehicle fire.
- Assess and triage each patient. Treat any life-threatening conditions.
- Reassess patients and provide stabilization and/or shock treatment until EMS arrives. (pages 451–452)

Skills

Skill Drills

Skill Drill 20-1: Accessing the Vehicle Through the Window
  1. Place the spring-loaded center punch at the **lower** corner of the **window**.
  2. Press the center punch to **break** the window.
  3. Remove the **glass** to the outside.
  4. Enter the **vehicle** through the **window**. (page 454)

Skill Drill 20-3: Turning a Patient in the Water
  1. Support the **back** and **head** with one hand. Place your other hand on the **front** of the patient.
  2. Carefully turn the patient as a **unit**.
  3. Stabilize the patient's **head** and **neck**. (page 459)

Chapter 21: Incident Management

General Knowledge

Matching

1. E (page 483)
2. H (page 484)
3. L (page 482)
4. D (page 483)
5. A (page 482)
6. K (page 482)
7. C (page 483)
8. N (page 479)
9. G (page 472)
10. O (page 485)
11. M (page 472)
12. I (page 482)
13. F (page 472)
14. B (page 485)
15. J (page 474)

Multiple Choice

1. D (page 483)
2. A (pages 485–486)
3. A (page 485)
4. D (page 479)
5. D (page 479)
6. B (pages 482–483)
7. C (page 483)
8. B (pages 479, 481)
9. C (page 485)
10. B (page 478)
11. D (page 471)
12. B (page 471)
13. A (page 473)
14. C (page 473)
15. A (page 474)
16. B (pages 474–475)
17. A (page 474)
18. C (page 475)
19. C (page 475)
20. D (page 477)
21. B (page 478)
22. A (page 478)

True/False

1. T (page 485)
2. T (page 485)
3. T (page 482)
4. F (page 483)
5. T (page 482)
6. F (page 482)
7. F (page 471)
8. T (page 475)
9. F (page 476)
10. F (page 482)

Crossword Puzzle

```
 1
 I
 N                 2              3
 C                 C              M
 U              4  S T A R T T R I A G E
 B                 S              S
 A          5      U        6     S            7
 T          I      A        W     C            E
 8 I N S E C T I C I D E S        A            X
 O          C      Y        M     U            P
 N        9 N I M S      10 H A Z A R D O U S  L
 P          E      O        L     L            O
 E                 R        T     T            S
 R       11 H O T Z O N E   Y     Y            I
 I                 I                           V
 O                 N                           E
 D                 G                           S
```

Critical Thinking

Fill-in-the-Blank

1. weapon; mass destruction (page 479)
2. explosive (page 482)
3. dosimeter (page 485)
4. biologic (page 484)
5. incubation (page 484)
6. START (page 476)
7. *Emergency Response Guidebook* (page 471)
8. hot zone (page 472)
9. urgent care (page 474)
10. gray; black (page 475)

Short Answer

1. 1. Pulmonary (choking) agents
   2. Metabolic agents
   3. Insecticides
   4. Nerve agents
   5. Blister agents (page 482)
2. Any three of the following:
   - Salivation
   - Sweating
   - Lacrimation (excessive tearing)

- Urination
- Defecation or diarrhea
- Gastric upset
- Emesis (vomiting) (page 483)

3. Nausea, vomiting, and diarrhea (page 485)

4. Any three of the following:
- Hospitals
- Research facilities
- Nuclear power plants
- Manufacturing sites for military weapons (page 485)

5. • Shortness of breath
- Flushed skin
- Rapid heartbeat
- Seizures
- Coma
- Cardiac arrest (pages 482–483)

6. **1.** Location of the incident
2. Type of incident
3. Any hazards
4. Approximate number of patients
5. Type of assistance required (page 473)

7. Simple Triage And Rapid Treatment (page 474)

8. **1.** Command and Management
2. Preparedness
3. Resource Management
4. Communications and Information Management
5. Supporting Technologies
6. Ongoing Management and Maintenance (page 478)

You Make the Call

1. Your answer should include the following steps and information:
- Carefully survey the scene for safety.
- Call for assistance from a specially trained hazardous materials response team.
- Establish an incident command system as soon as possible.
- Do not treat any patients who have come into direct contact with the powder until they have been decontaminated.
- Be sure to take proper standard precautions before treating patients. (pages 471–472, 484–485)

2. Your answer should include the following steps and information:
- Perform a visual survey of the entire scene before exiting your vehicle.
- Immediately identify any potential hazards and take the necessary precautions to make the scene safe for you, the patients, and the bystanders.
- Communicate the findings from your scene size-up to the communications center. Be specific in your request for additional help.
- Establish some form of an incident command until higher trained personnel arrive.
- Begin triaging patients using the START system, making sure you only stop to quickly correct airway and bleeding problems.
- Provide a verbal report to the EMS service arriving at the incident. (pages 473–478)